MCQs

in

MCQs in Orthodontics

K Vijayalakshmi
MDS
Dental Surgeon and Orthodontist
Professor and HOD of Orthodontics
Principal
JKK Nataraja Dental College
Komarapalayam, Namakkal Dt.
Tamil Nadu

JAYPEE BROTHERS
MEDICAL PUBLISHERS (P) LTD
New Delhi

Published by
Jitendar P Vij
Jaypee Brothers Medical Publishers (P) Ltd
EMCA House, 23/23B Ansari Road, Daryaganj
New Delhi 110 002, India
Phones: +91-11-23272143, +91-11-23272703, +91-11-23282021, +91-11-23245672
Fax: +91-11-23276490, +91-11-23245683 e-mail: jaypee@jaypeebrothers.com
Visit our website: www.jaypeebrothers.com

Branches

- 202 Batavia Chambers, 8 Kumara Krupa Road, Kumara Park East
Bangalore 560 001, Phones: +91-80-22285971, +91-80-22382956, +91-80-30614073
Tele Fax: +91-80-22281761 e-mail: jaypeebc@bgl.vsnl.net.in
- 282 IIIrd Floor, Khaleel Shirazi Estate, Fountain Plaza
Pantheon Road, **Chennai** 600 008, Phones: +91-44-28262665, +91-44-28269897
Fax: +91-44-28262331 e-mail: jpmedpub@md3.vsnl.net.in
- 4-2-1067/1-3, Ist Floor, Balaji Building, Ramkote
Cross Road, **Hyderabad** 500 095, Phones: +91-40-55610020, +91-40-24758498
Fax: +91-40-24758499 e-mail: jpmedpub@rediffmail.com
- 1A Indian Mirror Street, Wellington Square
Kolkata 700 013, Phone: +91-33-22451926 Fax: +91-33-22456075
e-mail: jpbcal@cal.vsnl.net.in
- 106 Amit Industrial Estate, 61 Dr SS Rao Road, Near MGM Hospital
Parel, **Mumbai** 400 012, Phones: +91-22-24124863, +91-22-24104532, +91-22-30926896
Fax: +91-22-24160828 e-mail: jpmedpub@bom7.vsnl.net.in

MCQs in Orthodontics

First Edition : **2006**

ISBN 81-8061-582-0

Typeset at JPBMP typesetting unit
Printed at Sanat Printers

to

My parents, my husband and my two children.

My Father	:	*Thiru S R Kuppuswamy*
My Mother	:	*Mrs K Krishnaveni*
My Husband	:	*Dr G Ravindran*
My First Son	:	*R Arun Jaikumar*
My Second Son	:	*R Pradeep Kumar*

J.K.K. Nataraja Dental College
KOMARAPALAYAM - 638 183, Namakkal Dt. Tamil Nadu. S. India

Mrs. N. SENDAMARAAI
Secretary
04288 - 260797

Prof. Dr. K.VIJAYALAKSHMI, MDS.,
Principal
04288 - 260203
04288 - 265793 (Fax)

Foreword

I am very happy to write a foreword for this book of *MCQs in Orthodontics* by Prof Dr K Vijayalakshmi MDS, Principal and Head of the Department of Orthodontics in our JKK Nataraja Dental College, Komarapalayam.

I congratulate Dr K Vijayalakshmi for all the efforts taken to bring out this book successfully, which is the result of her two years of continuous hard work.

I am sure that this book will be useful not only to the undergraduate and but to the postgraduate students also, for their study and reference.

I hope that the book will be overwhelmingly received and accepted with more edition to come with updated information on the subject in the rapidly changing world of Dental science.

Mrs N Sendamaraai
Secretary & Correspondent,
JKK Nataraja Educational Institutions,
Komarapalayam

Preface

With the help from the various contributors, I am able to compile and present nearly more than 700 MCQs including my own MCQs exclusively in Orthodontics. Since the Dental Science, technology, orthomaterials and appliances design are so advancing day by day and it is my duty to update the orthodontic knowledge to BDS students so that it will be fruitful to them in various PG entrance examinations.

Keeping this aspect in mind, I have listed all the MCQs in different titles and I hope this presentation is very simple and informative.

K Vijayalakshmi

Contents

1

Growth and Development

1. **Spheno-occipital synchondrosis closes at the age of:**
   A. 16 years
   B. 19 years
   C. 23 years
   D. 25 years

2. **The "V" principle of growth is best illustrated by the:**
   A. Nasal septum
   B. Mandibular ramus
   C. Mandibular symphysis
   D. Spheno-occipital synchondrosis

3. **The mandibular condyle grows by:**
   A. Endochondral bone formation
   B. Subperiosteal surface addition
   C. Interstitial growth
   D. Sutural bone growth

4. **Meckel's cartilage is essential for mandibular growth because:**
   A. It is converted into bone
   B. It is a template for bone deposition
   C. It is a skeletal unit
   D. It is a secondary cartilage

5. **The main growth site for mandible is:**
   A. Condyle
   B. Angle
   C. Symphysis
   D. Body

6. **The intercanine width in the mandible is completed by:**
   A. 4 to 5 years
   B. 7 to 8 years
   C. 9 to 10 years
   D. 10 to 12 years

---

1 D   2 B   3 A   4 B   5 A   6 C

7. **The condylar cartilage is a:**
   A. Primary cartilage
   B. Secondary cartilage
   C. Tertiary cartilage
   D. Septal cartilage

8. **Which of the following is a growth center?**
   A. Epiphyseal cartilage
   B. Condylar cartilage
   C. Sutures
   D. Symphysial cartilage

9. **The author of functional matrix theory is:**
   A. Melvin Moss
   B. Vander Linden
   C. Enlow
   D. Rolf Frankel

10. **At the cellular level, following are the possibilities for skeletal growth:**
    A. Hypertrophy
    B. Hyperplasia
    C. Secretion of extra-cellular material
    D. All of the above

11. **To understand growth in any area of the body, it is necessary to understand:**
    A. The sites or location of growth
    B. The type of growth occurring at that location
    C. Controlling factors in that growth
    D. All of the above

12. **Which of the following statements is correct regarding the size of the face at birth?**
    A. The face forms only 1/8th of the bulk of head, whereas in the adult it forms 1/3rd to 1/2 of the bulk
    B. The face forms 1/3rd the bulk of the head, whereas in the adult it forms 1/8th of the bulk
    C. The face forms 1/2 the bulk of the head throughout life
    D. The face forms 2/3rd the bulk of the head whereas in the adult it forms 1/3rd of the bulk

---

7 B 8 B 9 A 10 C 11 D 12 A

13. **According to functional matrix theory of Moss:**
    A. The growth of the skeletal components is largely dependent on growth of functional matrices
    B. Growth of functional matrices is largely dependent on the growth of skeletal components
    C. Growth of skeletal components is not dependent on the growth of functional matrices
    D. All of the above

14. **Which of the following statements is true?**
    A. All bones expand in 'V' shape producing opposition on inner aspect and resorption on external aspect
    B. Expansion of bones does not take place in 'V' shape
    C. All bones expand in 'V' shape producing resorption on inner aspect and apposition on external aspect
    D. None of the above

15. **The "safety valve" for correction of upper and lower basal bone discrepancy is:**
    A. Mandibular intercanine dimension
    B. Maxillary intercanine dimension
    C. Incisor liability
    D. Leeway space

16. **Which of the following methods is used for growth prediction?**
    A. Cephalometrics
    B. Handwrist X-rays
    C. Growth curves
    D. All of the above

17. **Which of the following are sites of cartilaginous growth postnatally?**
    i. Spheno-occipital synchondrosis
    ii. Frontomaxillary suture
    iii. Nasal septum
    iv. Alveolar process
    v. Condylar cartilage:
    A. i, iii and ii
    B. i, iii and v
    C. ii, iv and v
    D. All of the above

---

13 A 14 C 15 B 16 D 17 B

18. **In determining a patient's skeletal growth pattern, the most important factor is:**
    A. Diet
    B. Habits
    C. Heredity
    D. Dental occlusion

19. **Anterior cranial base becomes stable at about the age of:**
    A. 2 years
    B. 5 years
    C. 12 years
    D. 18 years

20. **Intermaxillary suture stops growing actively by the age of:**
    A. 6 to 18 months
    B. 4 to 5 years
    C. 7 to 9 years
    D. 12 to 14 years

21. **Out of the following growth is completed last at:**
    A. Calvarium
    B. Maxilla
    C. Nasion
    D. Mandible

22. **Which of the following sutures is the first to use?**
    A. Spheno-occipital
    B. Spheno-ethmoidal
    C. Intersphenoidal
    D. Interoccipital

23. **Spacing seen between the maxillary deciduous teeth in a 6-year old child indicates:**
    A. Good growth
    B. Class III tendency
    C. Class II tendency
    D. Presence of mesiodens

18 D 19 B 20 C 21 D 22 C 23 A

24. **After the age of 6 years, maximum growth of mandible is seen:**
A. Distal to the molars
B. In the area of the ramus
C. Symphyseal region
D. Mandible angle region

25. **The differential growth rate for different body tissues was described by:**
A. Scammon
B. Simon
C. Calvin S. Case
D. Norman William Kingsley

26. **Who defined as the growth is an increase in size, development is progress toward maturity?**
A. Todd
B. Graber
C. Krogman
D. Van der Linden

27. **When is the mandibular intercanine dimension completed in girls?**
A. 9 years
B. 10 years
C. 8 years
D. None of the above

28. **When is the mandibular intercanine dimension completed in boys?**
A. 10 years
B. 9 years
C. 12 years
D. 8 years

29. **When is the maxillary intercanine dimension completed in girls?**
A. 12 years B. 14 years
C. 18 years D. None of the above

24 A 25 A 26 A 27 A 28 A 29 A

30. When is the maxillary intercanine dimension completed in boys?

A. 18 years
B. 21 years
C. 14 years
D. 16 years

31. Which dimension in which arch is considered as a safety value for pubertal growth spurts?

A. Maxillary intercanine dimension
B. Mandibular intercanine dimension
C. Maxillary intermolar width
D. Mandibular intermolar width

32. Only intramembranous bone formation is for:

A. Mandible
B. Nasal
C. Temporal
D. Nasal conchae

33. Which of the following bone involves only intramembranous bone formation?

A. Mandible
B. Temporal
C. Ethmoid
D. Nasal

34. Maxilla articulates with all of the following bones *except:*

A. Frontal
B. Temporal
C. Zygomatic
D. Nasal

35. Maximum growth of the skull is completed by:

A. First 4 years of age
B. First 7 years of age
C. First 9 years of age
D. First 12 years of age

36. Maximum development of face takes place in:

A. 1st to 3rd week of IU life
B. 3rd to 8th week of IU life
C. 9th to 12th week of IU life
D. After 12th week of IU life

---

30 A 31 A 32 B 33 D 34 D 35 B 36 B

37. The initial sign of sexual maturation in boys usually is referred as:
- A. Fat spurt
- B. Growth spurt
- C. Onset of pubertal growth of spurt
- D. Peak growth

38. Which is responsible as primary cartilage for the growth of naso-maxillary complex?
- A. Nasal septum
- B. Septopremaxillary ligament
- C. Condylar cartilage
- D. None of the above

39. What is synchondrosis?
- A. A cartilaginous joint where the hyaline cartilage divides and subsequently is converted into bone
- B. This arrangement allows for a rapid increase in the length of the cranial base early in life to accommodate the growing brain
- C. Combination of A and B
- D. None of the above

40. Scammon growth curves includes:
- A. Four basic curves
- B. Five basic curves
- C. Six basic curves
- D. None of the above

41. Which is the longitudinal study?
- A. A study involves a large number of individuals of different ages are examined on one occasion to develop information.
- B. A study involves the examination of a group of children repeatedly over a long period during active growth.
- C. It presents in a graphic format, which reveals the substance of growth study findings in an easily grasped illustration.
- D. None of the above

37 A   38 A   39 C   40 A   41 B

42. **Which is cross-sectional study?**
   A. A study involves a large number of individuals of different ages are examined on one occasion to develop information.
   B. A study involves the examination of a group of children repeatedly over a long period during active growth.
   C. It presents in a graphic format, which reveals the substance of growth study findings in an easily grasped illustration.
   D. None of the above

43. **The late phase of childhood age ranges from:**
   A. 10 to 15 years
   B. 12 to 14 years
   C. 9 to 15 years
   D. 10 to 14 years

44. **The middle phase of childhood age ranges from:**
   A. 6 to 10 years
   B. 7 to 10 years
   C. 6 to 12 years
   D. 6 to 9 years

45. **Early phase of childhood age ranges from:**
   A. 1 to 6 years
   B. 2 to 6 years
   C. 1 to 7 years
   D. 1 to 5 years

46. **The childhood is divided into:**
   A. Three phase (early, middle and late phase)
   B. Two phase (early and late phase)
   C. Four phase (infancy, early, late and middle)
   D. None of the above

47. **Which period is called as infancy?**
   A. First year after birth
   B. Second year after birth
   C. Till 5 years
   D. All of the above

---

42 A 43 A 44 A 45 A 46 A 47 A

48. The adolescence period in girls starts from:
A. 10 to 20 years
B. 13 to 20 years
C. 14 to 20 years
D. None of the above

49. The adolescence period in boys starts from:
A. 14 to 20 years
B. 10 to 20 years
C. 10 to 25 years
D. Less than 20 years

50. The postnatal growth is comprised of:
A. Three period, infancy, childhood and adolescence
B. Two period, infancy, childhood
C. Throughout the growth stage after 25 years
D. None of the above

51. Postnatal growth is defined as:
A. The first 20 years of growth after birth
B. The first 25 years of growth after birth
C. The growth even at older ages
D. None of the above

52. First evidence of calcification of deciduous incisors is at:
A. 2 months
B. Between 1 to 2 months
C. 30 weeks *in utero*
D. 11 weeks *in utero*

53. The following statements are true:
A. Between the times when roots of the deciduous teeth have been completed with root resorption there is a 2 to 3 year rest period
B. Root resorption of deciduous teeth is not dependent on the presence of their permanent successor
C. In the permanent teeth, path of eruption is guided by the tubernaculum
D. A, B, C are true
E. Only A and C are true

---

48 B 49 A 50 A 51 A 52 D 53 D

54. **The maxillary second premolar erupts:**
  A. Straight occlusally
  B. Slightly buccally
  C. More often palatally
  D. In a transversely buccal path

55. **'First branchial arch' gives the following:**
  A. Maxilla
  B. Mandible, palate
  C. Zygomatic and squamous bones
  D. All of the above

56. **The two hemimandibles fuse at the symphysis at around:**
  A. 4 years of age
  B. 5 ½ months *in utero*
  C. 1 year of age
  D. Do not fuse as the union is fibrous

57. **Which of the following dental anomalies is usually not associated with cleft lip and palate?**
  A. Congenitally missing teeth
  B. Malposed teeth
  C. Supernumerary teeth
  D. Staining of teeth

58. **Early closure of a suture is called:**
  A. Synchondrosis
  B. Ankylosis
  C. Synostosis
  D. Epiphysis

59. **Clefting of the lip occurs because of failure of fusion between:**
  A. Median nasal process and lateral nasal process
  B. Frontal process and median nasal process
  C. Lateral nasal process and frontal process
  D. None of the above

---

54 C 55 D 56 C 57 D 58 A 59 A

60. **The structures of face are derived from:**
   A. Neural crest cells
   B. Phagocytic cells
   C. Osteoclast cell
   D. Haemocytis

61. **The child growth status is evaluated best by:**
   A. Biologic/developmental age
   B. Chronologic age
   C. Combination of A and B
   D. None of the above

62. **The localized bone growth problem can be diagnosed best by using:**
   A. Gamma emitting isotopes $99^{m}Tc$
   B. Tetracycline staining
   C. Alizarin
   D. All of the above

63. **The most common congenital defect involving face is:**
   A. Cleft lip
   B. Cleft palate
   C. Hemifacial microsomia
   D. Cliedo-cranial dysplasia

64. **All the orofacial muscles are:**
   A. Striated muscles
   B. Non-striated muscles
   C. Both striated and non-striated muscles
   D. None of the above

65. **Which of the following nerves is involved in troublesome gagger?**
   A. Glossopharyngeal nerve
   B. Trigeminal nerve
   C. Vagus nerve
   D. Both glossopharyngeal and trigeminal nerve

60 A 61 A 62 D 63 A 64 A 65 D

66. Except mandibular condyles, most of the mandibular growth is:
A. Intramembranous in nature
B. Endochondral in nature
C. Both intramembranous and endochondral in nature
D. None of the above

67. Which of the following is considered to be most stable of all of craniofacial skeleton structures?
A. Basicranium
B. Neurocranium
C. Cranial vault
D. Sphenoid bone

68. The growth mechanism of nasomaxillary complex involves:
A. Sutures only
B. Nasal septum
C. Endosteal and periosteal surface and alveolar process
D. All of the above

69. The development of tongue occurs during:
A. 2nd to 4th week of IUL
B. 4th to 6th week of IUL
C. 4th to 8th week of IUL
D. 6th to 10th week of IUL

70. Differentiation of human face occurs between:
A. 3rd and 5th week after fertilisation
B. 5th and 7th week after fertilisation
C. 7th and 9th week after fertilisation
D. 6th and 8th week after fertilisation

71. Most structures of adult face develop from:
A. First and second branchial arch and tissue surrounding the forebrain
B. 2nd and 3rd branchial arch and tissues surrounding the forebrain
C. 1st and 4th branchial arch
D. 1st and 3rd branchial arch

66 A 67 A 68 D 69 C 70 D 71 A

72. **The incidence of cleft lip and palate is:**
A. 1 in 600 B. 1 in 700
C. 1 in 800 D. 1 in 900

73. **The cleft lip defect appears most commonly during:**
A. 5th to 6th week
B. 6th to 7th week
C. 7th to 8th week
D. 4th to 5th week

74. **The skull at birth contains:**
A. 45 separated bones
B. 44 separated bones
C. 43 separated bones
D. 42 separated bones

75. **The adult skull contains:**
A. 20 bones
B. 21 bones
C. 22 bones
D. 23 bones

76. **The lower face appears at birth:**
A. Prognathic
B. Retrognathic
C. Straight
D. None of the above

77. **Premaxilla and maxilla appear from bilaterally located bony centres in anterior palate during:**
A. 7th week
B. 8th week
C. 9th week
D. 10th week

78. **The muscles of mastication develop in the mesenchyme of mandibular arch during:**
A. 5th week B. 6th week
C. 7th week D. 8th week

72 C 73 B 74 A 75 C 76 B 77 B 78 C

79. **In adult, the cranium to face ratio is:**
A. 4 : 1
B. 2 : 1
C. 1 : 2
D. 2 : 4

80. **The bony palate is very well established by the:**
A. 120°
B. 130°
C. 140°
D. 150°

81. **Which of the following mechanisms of bone growth is the predominant mode of growth in the skull?**
A. Endochondral ossification
B. Intramembranous ossification
C. Both intramembranous and endochondral ossification
D. None of the above

82. **The "Suture Dominance Theory" of craniofacial growth was given by:**
A. Moss
B. Sicher
C. Profitt
D. Petrovic

83. **Spurts in mandibular dimension are more frequently seen in:**
A. Boys than girls
B. Girls than boys
C. Both have same number of spurts in mandibular dimension
D. None of the above is correct

84. **From a clinical standing, the most significant overall sexual differences are seen in the achievement of:**
A. Facial length
B. Facial width
C. Facial height
D. None of the above

85. **Neonatal teeth:**
A. Present at the time of birth
B. Erupt during first month after birth
C. Erupt during 2nd/3rd month after birth
D. None of the above

---

79 B 80 C 81 B 82 B 83 A 84 C 85 B

86. Superimposition in longitudinal cephalometric studies are generally on a reference plane and a registration point. This best demonstrates the growth of:
A. Plane and point
B. Structures farthest from plane and point
C. Structures nearest to plane and point
D. All of the above

87. The sequence of completion of facial growth by planes of space is:
A. Depth, width, height
B. Height, depth, width
C. Width, depth, height
D. Depth, height, width

88. Supervision of a child's development of occlusion is most critical at age of:
A. 3 to 6 years
B. 7 to 10 years
C. 11 to 14 years
D. 14 to 17 years

89. The "V" principle of growth is best illustrated by the:
A. Nasal septum
B. Mandibular ramus
C. Mandibular symphysis
D. Spheno-occipital synchondrosis

90. The ossification centers of the mandible:
A. Are two in number and lateral to Meckel's cartilage
B. Are two in number and medial to Meckel's cartilage
C. Is one in number and lateral to Meckel's cartilage
D. Is one in number and medial to Meckel's cartilage

91. Most cranial sutures close by the age of:
A. 2 years
B. 3 years
C. 5 years
D. 8 years

86 B 87 C 88 B 89 B 90 A 91 C

92. **An early prepubertal growth spurt indicates:**
A. A longer treatment time
B. A fast maturing child
C. A slow maturing child
D. An endocrine dysfunction

93. **Ectodermal cells are responsible for:**
A. Alveolar bone
B. Periodontal tissue
C. Cementum formation
D. Determining crown and root shape

94. **Vertical growth of the face is attributed to growth at all sites *except:***
A. Frontonasal process of maxilla
B. Alveolar process of maxilla and mandible
C. Condylar process of mandible
D. Posterior border of ramus

95. **The mid-symphyseal suture fuses at the age of:**
A. 6 months
B. 18 months
C. 2 years
D. 5 years

96. **Premaxilla is derived from:**
A. Maxilla protuberance
B. Palatine bones
C. Frontonasal process
D. Median process

97. **Until the mature stage is attained, the occlusal plane with reference to a constant point Sella:**
A. Drops at the rate of 5 mm/year
B. Drops at the rate of 0.5 mm/year
C. Is elevated at the rate of 5 mm/year
D. Is elevated at the rate of 0.5 mm/year

92 B 93 D 94 D 95 B 96 C 97 B

98. **All of the following are active growth sites of the mandible, *except:***
A. Coronoid process
B. Alveolar process
C. Mandibular symphysis
D. Posterior border of the ramus
E. Condyle

99. **The downward and forward growth of the face is primarily the result of:**
A. Eruption of the teeth
B. Sutural growth of the skull
C. Growth of the maxillary sutures and the mandibular condyle
D. Interstitial growth in the maxilla and the mandible

100. **Relatively, the greatest dimension of the face at birth is:**
A. Width
B. Height
C. Depth
D. Any of the above

101. **The growth velocity reaches its peak in girls:**
A. 6 months ahead of boys
B. One year after that of boys
C. 2 years ahead of boys
D. At the same time as in boys

102. **The maxilla grows in width primarily by:**
A. Sutural growth
B. Subperiosteal growth
C. Endochondral growth
D. Endosteal growth

103. **All of the following are active growth sites of the maxilla, *except:***
A. Incisive foramen
B. Alveolar process
C. Tuberosity area
D. Midpalatal suture

98 C 99 C 100 A 101 C 102 A 103 A

104. As a child matures into an adult, what changes take place in the facial profile?

A. Facial profile flattens
B. The lips become more prominent as compared to the nose and chin
C. The face elongates and becomes narrower
D. There is no change in facial profile

105. By definition, growth may occur:

A. By both an increase in cell size and increase in cell number
B. By increase in cell size alone
C. By increase in cell size number alone
D. None of the above

106. To understand growth in any area of the body, it is necessary to understand:

A. The sites or location of growth
B. The type of growth occurring at that location
C. Controlling factors in that growth
D. All of the above

107. Growth changes can be studied and analyzed best by:

A. Patient history
B. Cephalometric radiographs
C. Diagnostic plaster casts
D. Bite wing radiographs
E. Observing siblings

108. The bony mandible develops as a thin, flat, rectangular bar:

A. Mesial to Meckel's cartilage
B. Lateral to Meckel's cartilage
C. Develops from condylar cartilage
D. Develops from sphenomandibular cartilage

---

104 A 105 A 106 D 107 B 108 B

109. **During growth of the maxilla and the mandible remodeling, resorption takes place on the nasal floor in the maxilla while in the mandible, it takes place on:**
   A. The alveolar process
   B. Posterior border of the ramus
   C. Anterior border of the ramus
   D. Mid symphysis

110. **Absence of the sesamoid bone at the average age of onset of puberty would mean:**
   A. Runs along the alveolar ridge to insert into the incisive papilla
   B. Is papery thin and thickens with age
   C. Is yet to develop
   D. Has a high attachment which is lowered with age

111. **At birth, which of the following structures is nearest to the size, it will eventually attain in adulthood?**
   A. Mandible
   B. Cranial vault
   C. Cranial base
   D. Middle face

---

109 C **110** C **111** B

2

Development of Dentition

1. **Mesial step formation in deciduous dentition is usually indication of a future:**
   A. Class II
   B. Class III
   C. Anterior crowding
   D. Anterior cross bite
2. **Arch length mesial to the first permanent mandibular molar, after the age of 6 years normally:**
   A. Remains nearly unchanged
   B. Increases
   C. Decreases
   D. No change
3. **According to Hay Nance the leeway space, which is used in the development of occlusion in maxillary and mandibular arch is ________ respectively:**
   A. 1.8 mm and 3.4 mm   B. 0.9 mm and 1.7 mm
   C. 2.3 mm and 1.4 mm   D. 1.2 mm and 1.9 mm
4. **A child aged 7½ years has a 2.5 mm midline diastema and partially erupted lateral incisor the parent should be advised that:**
   A. The condition should be corrected as it will hinder eruption of lateral incisor
   B. The condition is not abnormal for the age
   C. The condition is self-correcting but cannot be described as to why this has happened
   D. The lateral frenum should be dissected immediately

1 B   2 C   3 A   4 C

5. **In mixed dentition, which of the following may be considered as a self-correcting problem with age?**
   A. Unilateral loss of primary canine
   B. Lack of interdental spaces
   C. A distal step
   D. Open bite

6. **Order of eruption of permanent teeth in a maxillary arch is:**
   A. 6123457 B. 6124357
   C. 6124537 D. 43

7. **The change observed in the arch length of a child between 3 to 18 years is:**
   A. 4 mm B. 11 mm
   C. 17 mm D. 34 mm

8. **Occlusal adjustment is affected by all *except:***
   A. Compensating curve
   B. Cusp height
   C. Incisal guidance
   D. Postural position

9. **After eruption of teeth, root is completed within:**
   A. 1½ to 2½ years
   B. 2½ to 3½ years
   C. 5 to 6 years
   D. 5 to 6 months

10. **Intercanine width is increased with:**
    A. Eruption of lateral incisors
    B. Eruption of permanent canines
    C. Eruption of premolars
    D. Eruption of peg laterals

11. **The first tooth bud develops when embryo length is:**
    A. 6 mm B. 10 mm
    C. 12 mm D. 20 mm

5 C 6 C 7 A 8 D 9 B 10 B 11 A

12. In an ideal occlusion, which of the following is undesirable?
A. Crown angulation
B. Crown inclination
C. Curves of Spee
D. Spacing

13. Dental age is most closely related to:
A. Dental maturation
B. Resorption of roots
C. Diffuse calcification of pulp
D. Chronological age

14. Which of the following is a self-correcting anomaly?
A. Ugly duckling stage
B. Deep bite
C. Retrusion
D. Protrusion

15. Primate spaces in the primary dentition are seen between:
A. Maxillary central and lateral incisor and mandibular central incisor and canine
B. Maxillary primary first molar and second molar and mandibular canine and first primary molar
C. Maxillary primary lateral incisor and primary canine and mandibular primary canine and first primary molar
D. None of the above

16. Primate spaces are a characteristic of:
A. Most mammalian species
B. Human beings
C. Frogs
D. Cows and men

17. The leeway space is:
A. More in maxilla than in mandible
B. More in mandible than in maxilla
C. Equal in maxilla and mandible
D. None of the above

12 D 13 D 14 A 15 C 16 A 17 B

18. A distal step in the deciduous dentition leads to:
A. A normal relationship of permanent teeth
B. A class II malocclusion in permanent teeth
C. A class III malocclusion in permanent teeth
D. End to end relationship in permanent teeth

19. At what age is a child expected to have 12 erupted primary teeth and 12 erupted permanent teeth?
A. 4.5 years
B. 6.5 years
C. 8.5 years
D. 11.5 years

20. First permanent molars begin to calcify at:
A. 6 months of intrauterine life
B. At birth
C. Before deciduous incisors
D. About 1 year after birth

21. Before eruption, the position of permanent mandibular incisor buds relative to primary incisors is:
A. Superior and facial
B. Superior and lingual
C. Inferior and facial
D. Inferior and lingual

22. Tooth buds generally initiated after birth are:
A. The entire permanent dentition only
B. All permanent teeth and some primary teeth
C. First and second premolars and second and third molars only
D. All of the above

23. First evidence of calcification of 2nd premolar on radiographs is:
A. At birth
B. 3 to 4 months
C. 4 to 5 months
D. 1.5 to 2.5 years

18 B 19 C 20 B 21 D 22 C 23 D

24. **Apexogenesis is:**
   A. Formation of the apical one-third of the root
   B. Formation of the apical two-thirds of the root
   C. Closure of the apical foramen in a developing tooth
   D. Deposition of cellular cementum at the apex of the root

25. **During the transition from deciduous to permanent dentition, the overbite tends to decrease. This is mainly attributed to:**
   A. Change in axial inclination of permanent incisors
   B. Alveolar bone growth
   C. Physiologic bite opening
   D. All of the above

26. **Late mesial shift occurs due to:**
   A. Presence of Leeway space
   B. Primate spaces
   C. Presence of unrestored caries on distal surface of teeth
   D. In adults due to attrition of proximal surfaces of teeth

27. **Late mesial shift of mandibular permanent first molar is compensated by:**
   A. Primate spaces
   B. Median diastema
   C. Leeway space
   D. Wearing of proximal contacts of premolar teeth

28. **The calcification of the primary teeth begins about:**
   A. 11th week of IUL
   B. 12th week of IUL
   C. 14th week of IUL
   D. 16th week of IUL

29. **The time of initiation of first permanent molar formation *(in utero)*:**
   A. 2nd month
   B. 4th month
   C. 6th month
   D. 7th month

---

24 C 25 C 26 A 27 C 28 A 29 B

30. **According to Broadbent the "ugly duckling space" is the period from eruption of:**
    A. Central incisors to lateral incisors
    B. Lateral incisor to canine
    C. Canine to premolars
    D. Central incisor to canine

31. **Radiographs of the jaws of a newborn child ordinarily indicate calcification of:**
    A. 12 teeth
    B. 16 teeth
    C. 20 teeth
    D. 24 teeth

32. **Radiographs of a 5-year-old patient shows permanent maxillary first molars inclined mesially with resulting resorption of the distal portions of the roots of primary second molars. The condition described is:**
    A. Ankylosis
    B. Ectopic eruption
    C. Premature eruption
    D. Internal resorption

33. **Natural bite opener is the eruption of:**
    A. 6 years molar at the molar (first) eruption; later at the 2nd molar eruption
    B. Gives the picture of open bite
    C. During growing stages
    D. None of the above

30 A 31 D 32 B 33 A

3

Dental Occlusion and Stomatognathic System

1. **The teeth which are most often referred to as the key to normal occlusion are:**
   A. First permanent molars
   B. First permanent molars and second primary molars
   C. Maxillary and mandibular second primary molars
   D. Second permanent molars

2. **The six keys to normal occlusion was introduced by:**
   A. Dewey
   B. Andrews
   C. Tweed
   D. Angle

3. **The pharyngeal muscle which forms a part of buccinator mechanism is:**
   A. Inferior constrictor
   B. Middle constrictor
   C. Superior constrictor
   D. Palatopharyngeal

4. **Leeway space helps in the development of normal occlusion by:**
   A. Allowing mesial drift of molars
   B. Providing space for eruption of premolars
   C. Providing space for eruption of permanent second molars
   D. All of the above

---

1 A 2 B 3 C 4 D

5. **Which period is considered as late mixed dentition period?**
   A. Between 6 to 9 years
   B. Between 7 to 12 years
   C. Between 9 to 12 years
   D. Between 8 to 12 years

6. **The trajectorial theory of bone states that:**
   A. The bony trabeculae correspond to the pathways of maximum internal stress within the bone
   B. The bony trabeculae correspond to the lines of minimum internal stress within the bone
   C. The bony trabeculae are thin where the stress is greatest
   D. All of the above

7. **The "mandibular sling" consisting of the masseter and internal pterygoid muscles and the sphenomandibular ligament are responsible for establishing:**
   A. The physiologic rest position of the mandible
   B. The centric relation of the mandible in cooperation with other muscles of mastication
   C. The centric occlusion of the mandible
   D. All of the above

8. **During mastication pressures exerted on teeth range from:**
   A. 400 to 700 pounds
   B. 150 to 500 pounds
   C. 50 to 150 pounds
   D. Upto 1000 pounds

9. **Who put forth the concept "Law of orthogonality"?**
   A. Julius Wolff
   B. Roux
   C. Meyer
   D. Culmann

10. **Who propounded the trajectorial theory of bone formation?**
   A. An anatomist, Meyer
   B. Mathematician, Culmann
   C. Combination of A and B
   D. None of the above

---

5 C 6 A 7 D 8 B 9 A 10 C

11. What is Bennett movement?

A. In the lateral shift of the mandible the articular disk moves toward the side of the working bite

B. A muscle develops its maximum force when all of its fibers are repeatedly stimulated to fire

C. The intensity of the contraction of any fiber is independent of the strength of the exciting stimulus, provided that the stimulus is adequate

D. None of the above

12. Who divided the deglutitional cycle into 4 phases?

A. Fletcher

B. Meyer

C. Benninghoff

D. Enlow

13. The instrument most often used for evaluating the activity of orofacial muscles:

A. Electromyograph

B. Holograph

C. Bronchoscope

D. Tonometer

14. Kinesiology is the study of movement resulting from action of:

A. Muscles

B. Nerve

C. Blood vessel

D. Cells

15. Which period is considered as early mixed dentition period:

A. Between 6 to 9 years

B. Between 7 to 12 years

C. Between 9 to 12 years

D. Between 8 to 12 years

---

11 A 12 A 13 A 14 A 15 A

4

Diagnosis, Classification of Malocclusion, Model and Cephalometric Analysis

DIAGNOSIS

1. **Brachycephalic individuals usually have:**
   A. Narrow dental arches
   B. Broad dental arches
   C. Normal dental arches
   D. B or C

2. **Carpel index denotes:**
   A. Number of carpal bones
   B. Skeletal maturity
   C. Treatment prognosis
   D. Incidence of malocclusion

3. **The best time to correct anteroposterior discrepancy in skeletal base is:**
   A. Primary dentition period
   B. Mixed dentition period
   C. Permanent dentition period
   D. Post-permanent dentition period

4. **Skeletal indicators of maturity are determined by:**
   A. Chest X-ray
   B. Periapical X-ray
   C. Hand wrist X-ray
   D. Occlusal X-ray
   E. Combination of B and C

---

1 B 2 B 3 B 4 E

5. **Total mandibular arch contained in maxillary arch is:**
   A. Scissors bite
   B. Deep bite
   C. Reverse bite
   D. Cross bite

6. **The facial profile in adenoid faces (mouth breathers) is characterized by:**
   A. Long and wide
   B. Long and narrow
   C. Short and wide
   D. Short and narrow

7. **Physio-print is a term used to describe:**
   A. Facial masks of patients taken before and after treatment
   B. A test to assess mental growth and correlate to dental growth
   C. A photographic orientation technique that permits measurements of facial contours and volumes
   D. Physiological assessment of growth changes

8. **The need for orthodontic treatment may arise for the following reasons:**
   A. To improve the physical appearance
   B. To reduce the chances of trauma
   C. As an adjunct in periodontal treatment
   D. All of the above

9. **Scissors bite may be defined as:**
   A. When upper arch lie palatal to the lower arch
   B. Edge to edge relation of upper and lower arch
   C. When upper arch teeth lie further buccally than their normal position
   D. Anterior cross bite

10. **Lip incompetency may be due to:**
    A. Increased anterior lower facial height
    B. Short resting lip length
    C. Large anteroposterior skeletal discrepancy usually class II malocclusion
    D. All of the above

---

5 A 6 B 7 C 8 D 9 C 10 D

11. The most difficult malocclusion to be corrected by orthodontic treatment is:
A. Class II division 2
B. Class III with horizontal growth pattern
C. Class III with vertical growth pattern
D. Bimaxillary protrusion

12. The ideal proportion of upper facial height to lower facial height is:
A. 45% : 55%
B. 55% : 45%
C. 40% : 60%
D. 50% : 50%

13. The anterior lower facial height is decreased in:
A. Skeletal open bite
B. Skeletal deep bite
C. Long face syndrome
D. Backward rotating mandible

14. Dental arch form is ultimately determined by the:
A. Facial type
B. Angle classification
C. Facial growth pattern
D. Balance between facial and intraoral musculature
E. Interaction of environmental influence on the genetic pattern

15. Most class III malocclusions are associated with:
A. Skeletal class III pattern
B. Deep bites
C. Open bite
D. Competent lips

16. Overclosure of the mandible occurs when there is extensive loss of posterior teeth. This can lead to:
A. Clicking of temporomandibular joint
B. Destruction of the articular disk
C. Crepitus
D. None of above

11 C 12 A 13 B 14 E 15 A 16 B

17. **Which of the following is not true?**
    A. Deep bite is often associated with maxillary prognathism
    B. Open bite is associated with an increase in anterior facial height
    C. Mandibular prognathism is less common than maxillary prognathism
    D. Myofunctional therapy is indicated for tongue thrusting

18. **A large overjet may be caused by:**
    A. Maxillary prognathism
    B. Retrognathic mandible
    C. Lip biting
    D. All of the above

19. **In skeletal class III malocclusion, the speech difficulties will involve:**
    A. Labiodental fricative/f/v
    B. /S/z/(sibilants)
    C. /t/,/d/linguoalveolar stops
    D. th, sh, ch (linup-dental frication)

20. **The primary second molar teeth has a normal relationship in the form of:**
    A. Flush terminal plane
    B. Mesial step relationship
    C. Distal step relationship
    D. None of the above

21. **For future growth prediction, the visualized treatment objective (VTO) as a treatment planning tool in addition to the routine diagnostic methods was introduced first by:**
    A. Rickett's
    B. Steiner
    C. Holdaways
    D. Down's

---

17 D 18 A 19 A 20 A 21 A

22. **For good facial aesthetics, it is important to have:**
   - A. Correct maxillary midline
   - B. Correct mandibular midline
   - C. A slight displacement of mandibular midline
   - D. Correct maxillary and mandibular midline which corresponds to each other and with mid-sagittal plane

23. **Dental arch form is ultimately determined by:**
   - A. Facial type coupled with body type
   - B. Skeletal growth pattern
   - C. The functional relationship of the posterior teeth
   - D. Interaction of environmental influençe on the genetic pattern

24. **To localize a supernumerary or an impacted tooth and its exact relationship to other teeth, which of the following radiographs would be most effective?**
   - A. A periapical and an occlusal view
   - B. An occlusal view with a high angle
   - C. A panoramic X-ray with a supplemental periapical film
   - D. Two or more periapical views at different angles and an occlusal view

25. **A concave profile would reveal angle of convexity to be:**
   - A. Positive
   - B. Negative
   - C. 0°
   - D. Not predictable

26. **The vertical height of mandibular ramus is most accurately indicated by:**
   - A. Facial angle
   - B. Mandibular plane angle
   - C. Y axis
   - D. SNB angle

22 D 23 D 24 D 25 B 26 B

27. **In the treatment of traumatic intrusion it will be useless to:**
    A. Splint the tooth
    B. Take an X-ray
    C. Wait for its re-eruption
    D. Recall the patient

28. **Soft-tissue profile of a thumb sucking patient is:**
    A. Convex
    B. Concave
    C. Normal
    D. Anteriorly divergent

29. **A 14-year-old boy with operated cleft lip will have:**
    A. Maxillary protrusion
    B. Posterior arch cross bite
    C. Mandibular protrusion
    D. Maxillary retrusion

30. **On radiological examination, marked overlapping of developing permanent upper incisors denotes:**
    A. Severe crowding
    B. Normal growth
    C. Incisor liability helps the situation
    D. None of the above

31. **Which law is related to orthodontics?**
    A. Wolff's Law
    B. Newton's Law
    C. Canine Law
    D. All of the above

32. **Who carried the implant growth study?**
    A. Bjork
    B. Ricketts
    C. Steiners
    D. Tweed

---

27 A 28 A 29 D 30 A 31 D 32 A

33. If there is no physiological spacing in between deciduous incisors, what is your investigation?

A. Intra-oral X-ray periapical view
B. Study model
C. Cephalogram
D. All of the above

34. What is the importance of VTO (Visualized treatment objective) in orthodontics?

A. As a clinical diagnostic aid to select a case for functional appliance
B. As a superimposition technique
C. As a soft tissue analysis
D. None of the above

35. Which VTO is required for functional appliance?

A. +ve VTO
B. -ve VTO
C. Difficult to elicit
D. None of the above

36. Which type of malocclusion is most often associated with fractured maxillary anterior tooth?

A. Class I
B. Class II div 1
C. Class II div 2
D. Class III

37. Apertognathia is:

A. Anterior cross bite
B. Open bite
C. Posterior cross bite
D. Prognathism

38. Difference between dental open bite and skeletal open bite is:

A. In dental, open bite present from canine to canine whereas in skeletal, open bite presents from 1st premolar to 1st premolar
B. Dental open bite can be corrected orthodontically whereas skeletal open bite by functional appliance in young age or by surgical orthodontics
C. Both are same (A and B)
D. None of A and B

33 A 34 A 35 A 36 B 37 B 38 C

39. **Which is the supplemental diagnostic aid?**
 A. Study cost
 B. Facial photographs
 C. Cephalogram
 D. Clinical examination

40. **Appearance of sesamoid bone denotes:**
 A. Retardation of pubertal development
 B. Onset of puberty
 C. Peak growth
 D. No significance

41. **Initial ossification of the sesamoid and advanced ossification of the hook of the hamate denotes:**
 A. Peak growth
 B. Onset of puberty
 C. Decline of growth
 D. No significance

42. **When hand-wrist radiograph is not available what could be the other alternative to assess the pubertal growth spurt in your daily practice?**
 A. Periapical intra-oral mandibular radiograph
 B. Orthopantogram
 C. Cephalogram
 D. Bite wing films

43. **Root completion of lower left canine denotes:**
 A. Decline of pubertal growth
 B. Onset of puberty
 C. Peak growth
 D. Cessation of pubertal growth

44. **Which is the indicator of pubertal growth spurt?**
 A. Sesamoid bone and hook of Hamate
 B. Cervical vertebra
 C. Left lower canine
 D. All of the above

---

39 C 40 B 41 A 42 A 43 D 44 D

45. Overjet is the:
A. Horizontal overlap
B. Vertical overlap
C. Discrepancy in the transverse plane
D. None of the above

46. An Angle Class-II malocclusion is worsened by:
A. Overclosure
B. Short facial height
C. Decreased mandibular growth
D. Decreased lip activity

47. Fractured maxillary teeth generally occur most often in children with:
A. Maxillary retrusion
B. Class I malocclusion
C. Class II div. 1 malocclusion
D. Class II div. 2 malocclusion

48. In the context of orthodontics, morphology means:
A. Behaviour during function
B. Shape and size
C. Relationship
D. Development

49. A cross bite is dental malformation in:
A. Vertical plane
B. Antero-posterior plane
C. Transverse plane
D. All of the above

50. A square shaped arch is seen in which malocclusion:
A. Angle's Class I type
B. Angle's Class II div 1
C. Angle's Class II div. 2
D. Angle's Class III

---

45 A 46 C 47 C 48 B 49 C 50 C

51. **In a skeletal class III malocclusion, the mandible would have undergone a:**
   A. Backward rotation
   B. Forward rotation
   C. Clockwise rotation
   D. Distal rotation

52. **A patient with vertical growth tendency will have:**
   A. A Class III malocclusion
   B. Increased steepness of mandibular plane
   C. Palatal plane tipping downwards anteriorly
   D. Forward rotation of the mandible

53. **The tonicity of the upper lip in a mouth breather is:**
   A. Increased
   B. Decreased
   C. Not affected
   D. Any of the above

54. **The unfavourable sequelae of malocclusion can be:**
   A. Poor appearance
   B. Abnormal muscle function
   C. Predisposition to dental caries
   D. All of the above

55. **TMJ problems can arise due to malocclusion in the following manner:**
   A. Occlusal prematurities lead to TMJ trauma
   B. Deep bite predisposes to TMJ trauma
   C. Anterior cross bite with prognathic mandible results in TMJ trauma
   D. All of the above

56. **Chronological age of a child is:**
   A. Related to dental age
   B. Related to skeletal age
   C. Independent of dental or skeletal age
   D. Independent of dental age only but related to skeletal age

---

51 B 52 B 53 B 54 D 55 D 56 A

57. **Space closure is rapid following loss of which primary molars:**
   A. Maxillary molars; closing within three months
   B. Mandibular molars; closing within six months
   C. Maxillary molars; closing within six months
   D. Mandibular molars; closing within three months

58. **Deep skeletal bite will show which of the following features?**
   A. High mandibular plane
   B. Low mandibular plane
   C. Deep palate
   D. All of the above

59. **The two finger method of finding skeletal pattern is proposed by:**
   A. Mills
   B. Korkaus
   C. Jacobson
   D. Houstan

60. **Mirror technique is advocated to check:**
   A. Mouth breathing
   B. Nasal airway technique
   C. None of the above
   D. Combination of 1 and 2

61. **Which type of mirror is used in mirror technique to elicit mouthbreather?**
   A. Two surfaced steel mirror
   B. One surfaced mirror
   C. Concave mirror
   D. None of the above

62. **Who described the patients into Ectomorphic, endomorphic and mesomorphic?**
   A. Sheldon B. Graber
   C. Mills D. Profitt

57 D 58 B 59 A 60 D 61 A 62 A

63. **Arch expansion after appliance therapy is detected by:**
   A. Occlusal film
   B. Intraoral film
   C. Cephalogram
   D. A-P view

64. **Phonetic exercises are:**
   A. Reciting the letter 'M'
   B. Spelling the word "Mississippi'
   C. Combination of A and B
   D. None of A and B

65. **The patient has no idea of what is being examined as the patient voluntarily talk and swallows. This is a:**
   A. Non-command method of assessing of the postural rest position
   B. Command method
   C. Combined method
   D. None of the above

66. **One of the methods of assessing the postural rest position is:**
   A. Command method
   B. Two fingers method
   C. Butterfly technique
   D. Lip exercises

67. **Which is used to find the arch symmetry?**
   A. Symmetrograph
   B. With the help of fine divider
   C. Combination of both
   D. None of the above

68. **An anatomic cross bite, as contrasted with a functional cross bite, usually demonstrates:**
   A. Marked wear facets
   B. Smooth closure to centric occlusion
   C. Deviated closure to centric occlusion
   D. Symmetrical individual dental arches

---

63 A 64 C 65 A 66 A 67 A 68 B

69. **Surgery on the hard palate of a 3-year-old cleft patient may inhibit growth centers, causing the facial profile to become:**
    A. Straight
    B. Elongated
    C. More convex
    D. More concave

70. **The changes taking place in the facial profile with age are:**
    A. Profile becomes more concave
    B. Profile becomes more convex
    C. Flattening of profile takes place
    D. Any of the above

71. **Hand and wrist X-rays predict:**
    A. Timing of growth
    B. Direction of growth
    C. Amount of growth
    D. All of the above

72. **Facial photographs will not predict:**
    A. Profile
    B. Lip competency
    C. Chin prominence
    D. Anterior cross bite

73. **A patient with achondroplasia presents with:**
    A. Class I malocclusion
    B. Class II malocclusion
    C. Class III malocclusion
    D. None of the above

74. **A patient wearing Milwaukee's brace for the treatment of scoliosis may have:**
    A. Class III malocclusion
    B. Class I type 2 malocclusion
    C. Decreased vertical flap face height
    D. Proclined lower anteriors

---

69 D 70 C 71 A 72 D 73 C 74 C

75. **Labioversion of incisors may lead to:**
A. Gingival hypertrophy
B. Fibrosis of gingiva
C. Gingival inflammation
D. Any of the above

76. **Dolicocephalic patient has:**
A. Long, wide arches
B. Long, narrow arches
C. Short, wide arches
D. Short, narrow arches

77. **The malocclusion which can be prevented is:**
A. Loss of proximal contacts
B. Absence of teeth
C. Cleft palate
D. Endocrine disorder

78. **Primary teeth differ from permanent teeth in the following aspects:**
A. Thickness of enamel and dentin
B. Pulp chambers are longer
C. Roots are flaring
D. All of the above

79. **A malocclusion is characterized by contraction of maxillary denture, labioversion of maxillary incisors, deep over bite and over jet. These are typical characteristics of a malocclusion of which of the following Angle classification?**
A. Class-I
B. Class-II division 1
C. Class-II division 2
D. Class-III

80. **Severely crowded mandibular incisors usually result from:**
A. Mesial migration of teeth
B. Premature loss of primary teeth
C. Presence of supernumerary teeth
D. Tooth size arch length discrepancy

75 C 76 B 77 A 78 D 79 B 80 D

81. With a flush terminal plane, permanent first molars will:
A. Initially be class-II
B. Initially be class-III
C. Immediately assume a normal relationship
D. Erupt immediately into an end to end relationship

82. Which of the following factors may contribute to the severity of the incisor overbite in Class-II division 2 malocclusion?
A. Lip activity
B. Overclosure
C. The anteroposterior base relationship
D. The reduced lower face height

83. The anterior oral seal is:
A. Between roof of the tongue and vault of the palate
B. The approximation of upper and lower lips when the muscles (perioral) are relaxed
C. Between the root of the tongue and the soft palate
D. None of the above

84. The middle oral seal is:
A. Between roof of the tongue and vault of the palate
B. Between the root of the tongue and the soft palate
C. None of the above
D. All of the above

85. The posterior oral seal is:
A. Between the roof of the tongue and the soft palate
B. The tip of the tongue lies palatal to the upper incisors
C. All of the above
D. None of the above

---

81 D 82 C 83 B 84 A 85 A

CLASSIFICATION OF MALOCCLUSION

86. Which of the following condition is always present in Class II div 2 malocclusion?

A. Open bite
B. Cross bite
C. Deep bite
D. Closed bite

87. The major criteria to differentiate between a true class III and a pseudo class III malocclusion is:

A. Existence of a forward shift of the mandible during closure
B. Occlusal relationship between maxillary and mandibular first molar
C. Presence of posterior crossbite
D. Presence of anterior crossbite

88. Law of canine was proposed by:

A. Angle
B. Simon
C. Ackerman-Profit
D. Moss

89. A classification which is based on anatomical planes is:

A. Angle's classification
B. Simon's classification
C. Ackerman-Profitt classification
D. Lischer's classification

90. A premolar erupting in the place of the canine, it is said to be:

A. Torsiversion
B. Perversion
C. Transiversion
D. Mesioversion

91. Edward Hartley Angle is the contributor of:

A. Angle's classification
B. Edgewise appliance
C. All of the above (A and B)
D. None of the above

---

86 D 87 A 88 B 89 B 90 C 91 C

92. **A pseudo class III malocclusion is always associated with:**
   A. Deep bite
   B. Maxillary protrusion
   C. Maxillary retrusion
   D. Anterior cross bite

93. **Lips that are full and everted are usually associated with:**
   A. Retroclined upper and lower anterior teeth
   B. Proclined upper and lower anterior teeth
   C. Proclined upper and retroclined lower anterior teeth
   D. Retroclined upper and proclined lower anterior teeth

94. **A large freeway space is related to:**
   A. An increased overjet
   B. Anterior cross bite
   C. Posterior cross bite
   D. Anterior deep bite

95. **Hyperactivity of the mentalis muscle is generally observed in:**
   A. Class II division 1 malocclusion
   B. Class II division 2 malocclusion
   C. Class III malocclusion
   D. Class I malocclusion

96. **Gnathostatic model by Simon are those in which:**
   A. Base of the lower model corresponds to the FHP
   B. Base of the upper model corresponds to the FHP
   C. Base of the upper model corresponds to S-N plane
   D. Base of the lower model corresponds to S-N plane

97. **A tooth that, in vertical approach has not erupted to the line of occlusion is in:**
   A. Infraversion
   B. Supraversion
   C. Torsiversion
   D. Distoversion

---

92 D 93 C 94 D 95 A 96 B 97 A

98. Angle's classification of malocclusion is based on which of the following principles?

A. The most indicative irregularity of the teeth is in the anteroposterior direction

B. The maxillary first permanent molar is the key to occlusion

C. The curvature and size of the "line of occlusion" (greatest normal occlusal contact) is unique to each individual

D. None of the above

E. A, B and C are all correct

99. The terms "neutrocclusion" for Angle's class I "distocclusion" for class II and "mesiocclusion" for class III were suggested by:

A. Dewey Anderson

B. Angle himself later suggested these terms to simplify his classification

C. Lischer

D. Simon

100. The term "incompetent lips" refers to:

A. Lips which do not seal when relaxed with the mandible in its rest position

B. Lips against which tongue thrusts during swallowing

C. Lips that contract during swallowing

D. Lips which have some dryness in the divisions

101. The divisions in Angle's class I were proposed by:

A. Paul Simon

B. Martin Dewey

C. Edward H. Angle

D. Profitt

102. The skeletal classification of malocclusion was given by:

A. Calvin Case

B. Martin Dewey

C. Paul Simon

D. EH Angle

98 B 99 C 100 A 101 B 102 C

103. The Angles classification of malocclusion was given in:
A. 1888 B. 1889
C. 1890 D. 1891

104. The most prevalent form of malocclusion:
A. Angles class I malocclusion
B. Class II div. 1 malocclusion
C. Class II div. 2 malocclusion
D. Class III malocclusion

105. A convex facial profile is associated with:
A. Class I Jaw relationship
B. Class II Jaw relationship
C. Class III Jaw relationship
D. None of the above

106. The "Gnathostatic" system of classification of malocclusion was given by (1930):
A. Edward H. Angle
B. Calvin Case
C. Martin Dewey
D. Simon

107. Three dimensional classification occlusion was given by:
A. Angle B. Simon
C. Dewey D. Baume

108. When the occlusal plane closer to FHP it is called:
A. Abstraction
B. Contraction
C. Attraction
D. Protraction

109. The classification using deciduous 2nd molar was given by:
A. Angle B. Tweed
C. Baume D. Simon

103 C 104 A 105 B 106 D 107 B 108 C 109 B

110. Edward Hartley Angle was born in:
A. 1855
B. 1889
C. 1839
D. 1840

111. Who coined the term "the orthodontia"?
A. LeFoulon in 1839
B. Pierre Fauchard in 1725
C. Edward Hartley Angle in 1887
D. None of the above

112. The name orthodontics is derived from the following words:
A. Greek word
B. Latin word
C. American word
D. None of the above

113. Which year the BSO definition of orthodontics was proposed?
A. 1922
B. 1911
C. 1907
D. 1920

114. When the Angle's classification of malocclusion was published?
A. 1890
B. 1889
C. 1835
D. 1870

115. If the lower permanent molars are missing in permanent dentition, what is the other classification you select?
A. Canine classification
B. Incisor classification
C. Combination of A and B
D. None of the above

---

110 A 111 A 112 A 113 A 114 A 115 C

116. Which classification shows edge to edge bite?
- A. Cl-III malocclusion of dental type
- B. Pseudo Cl-III
- C. Skeletal Cl-III type
- D. None of the above

117. In Angle's class III malocclusion, mandibular anterior teeth will be:
- A. Proclined
- B. Retroclined
- C. Inclined
- D. Any of the above

118. In which malocclusion, maxillary incisor inclination is most vertical:
- A. Angle's class I, type II
- B. Angle's Class II, div I
- C. Angle's Class III
- D. None of the above

119. In Angle's class I malocclusion which of the following is not usual?
- A. Bimaxillary protrusion
- B. Rotation and crowding
- C. Closed bite
- D. All of the above

120. Functional retrusion may be seen in which malocclusion:
- A. Angle's class I
- B. Angle's class II div 2
- C. Angle's class III
- D. Any of the above

121. Angle class II malocclusions occur:
- A. Rarely
- B. In about 22 percent of the population
- C. In almost 50 percent of the population
- D. In more than 75 percent of the population

---

116 A 117 B 118 C 119 C 120 B 121 B

122. A disto-occlusion corresponds to:

A. Angle's Class I B. Angle's Class II
C. Angle's Class III D. None of the above

123. In Angle's Class I malocclusion:

A. Distal slope of maxillary canine overlaps distal slope of mandibular canine
B. Mesial slope of maxillary canine overlaps distal slope of mandibular canine
C. Mesial slope of maxillary canine overlaps mesial slope of mandibular canine
D. Distal slope of maxillary canine overlaps mesial slope of mandibular canine

124. A Gnathostatic approach:

A. Assumes Gnathion to be a stable landmark on a cephalogram
B. Is used to orient plaster study models on the patient's face
C. Eliminates the use of plaster study models to evaluate the position of occlusal plane
D. Uses Gnathion-Gonion plane as a plane of superimposition

125. Angle's classification is based on which tooth as stable landmark and guideline for occlusion:

A. Maxillary first permanent molar
B. Mandibular first permanent molar
C. Maxillary second permanent molar
D. Mandibular second permanent molar

126. Malocclusion is classified according to Angle considering the irregularity of teeth in the:

A. Anteroposterior plane
B. Lateral direction
C. Vertical plane
D. Transverse plane

122 B 123 B 124 C 125 A 126 A

127. Most of the cases of malocclusion fall under Angle's:

A. Class I
B. Class II
C. Class III
D. Class IV

128. Classification based on anthropological planes utilises:

A. Frankfurt Horizontal plane
B. Median sagittal plane
C. Orbital plane
D. All of the above

129. Which of the following is used in mixed dentition classification of malocclusion?

A. Flush terminal plane
B. Angle's classification
C. Simon's orbital plane
D. All of the above

130. Angle class II malocclusions occur:

A. Rarely
B. In about 22 percent of the population
C. In almost 50 percent of the population
D. In more than 75 percent of the population

131. Inability to pronounce bilabial consonants and a production of a lisp-like sound is associated with which type of malocclusion?

A. Class I with anterior cross bite
B. Class III
C. Class I with posterior cross bite
D. Class II div.1 with incompetent lips

132. A term to indicate the placement of teeth too far forward in the maxilla is:

A. Retroversion
B. Anteversion
C. Retraction
D. Supraversion

---

127 A 128 D 129 A 130 B 131 D 132 B

133. A term to indicate the placement of teeth too far away from the midline in an arch is:

A. Extraversion B. Retroversion
C. Contraction D. Infraversion

134. When a tooth is impacted, the condition is known as:

A. Transposition
B. Torsiversion
C. Perversion
D. Axiversion

135. When a tooth is rotated, the condition is known as:

A. Transposition
B. Torsiversion
C. Perversion
D. Axiversion

136. If the teeth are placed behind the orbital plane, the term used is:

A. Attraction B. Abstraction
C. Protraction D. Retraction

137. According to Simon, in most of the cases the orbital plane passes through:

A. Maxillary premolars
B. Maxillary canine
C. Mandibular canine
D. Mandibular canine

138. According to Simon, if the teeth are placed closer to a plane, the term used is "contraction" and if they are placed away, the term used is "distraction." These terms are used for the plane:

A. Frankfurt Horizontal plane
B. Median sagittal plane
C. Orbital plane
D. All of the above

133 A 134 C 135 B 136 D 137 B 138 B

139. Torsiversion is:
- **A.** Rotation of tooth around its own axis
- **B.** Fusion of cementum
- **C.** Rotation in horizontal direction
- **D.** None of the above

140. In mixed dentition analysis, which tooth is used for classification:
- **A.** Primary 1st molar
- **B.** Primary 2nd molar
- **C.** Permanent 1st molar
- **D.** B or C

141. Lower left first permanent molar is assigned no. 36 as per the formula of:
- **A.** FDI
- **B.** ADA
- **C.** IDA
- **D.** WHO

142. Symptomatic classification is a term used to describe:
- **A.** Dental malocclusion
- **B.** Skeletal malocclusion
- **C.** Functional malocclusion
- **D.** All of the above

143. In Angle's Class-I malocclusion which of the following is not seen?
- **A.** Cross bite
- **B.** Bimaxillary protrusion
- **C.** Occlusal surface of mandibular teeth overlaps the buccal surface of maxillary teeth
- **D.** Rotation and crowding

144. When Cl-II relationship is present on one side only and there is Class-I relationship on the otherside, it is called:
- **A.** Cl-II div 1
- **B.** Cl-II div 2
- **C.** Cl-II subdivision
- **D.** All of the above

139 A 140 C 141 A 142 D 143 C 144 C

145. Unilateral Cl-III molar relationship, with molars on the other side in Cl-I relationship is:

A. Cl-III div 1
B. Cl-III div 2
C. Cl-III subdivision
D. Any of the above

146. Angle's Cl-I and Cl-III have been categorized into different types by:

A. Lischer
B. Deway
C. Simon
D. Angle

147. Who termed malocclusion?

A. Guilford
B. Edward Hartley Angle
C. Deway
D. Simon

148. Who described six keys to normal occlusion?

A. Andrews
B. Begg
C. Bennett
D. Wick Alexander

MODEL ANALYSIS

149. A deficiency of 6-8 mm usually requires extraction of:

A. First molars
B. Second premolars
C. First premolars
D. Second molars

150. Howe's analysis helps in knowing:

A. Maxillo-mandibular relations
B. Basal bone tooth material discrepancy
C. Growth prediction
D. Age of the patient

---

145 C 146 B 147 A 148 A 149 C 150 B

151. Pont's analysis indicates:
A. Crowding in the upper arch
B. Constriction in the upper arch
C. Crowding in the lower arch
D. Constriction in the lower arch

152. Carey's analysis is done to find out:
A. Skeletal discrepancies in the upper arch
B. Space discrepancies in the lower arch
C. Transverse discrepancies in the upper arch
D. Space discrepancies in the upper arch

153. Bolton analysis is used for:
A. Analysing the tooth size discrepancies
B. Calculating anchorage values
C. Forecasting growth
D. Predicting prognosis

154. Which of the following cast analysis is done in permanent dentition?
A. Moyers analysis
B. Hixon and Oldfather's analysis
C. Carey's analysis
D. Huckaba's analysis

155. Peck and Peck index denotes:
A. The ratio of labiolingual to mesiodistal dimension of the mandibular canine
B. The ratio of labiolingual to mesiodistal dimension of the mandibular incisors
C. The ratio of cervico-incisal to mesiodistal dimension of the mandibular incisors
D. All of the above

156. Which of the following model analyses is used to determine discrepancy in the transverse direction?
A. Pont's index
B. Carey's analysis
C. Nance analysis
D. Peck and Peck analysis

151 B 152 B 153 A 154 C 155 B 156 A

157. **Which of the following had developed the methods to determine the size of unerupted teeth?**
A. Huckaba B. Nance
C. Moyers D. All of the above

158. **Moyers has given a table by which the size of unerupted (permanent) teeth may be predicted. In order to use this chart, we must know:**
A. The incisal lengths 21 12
B. The date of eruption of 21 12
C. The mesiodistal width of 21 12
D. The mesiodistal width of 6 6

159. **Which of the following methods of space analysis does not require use of either radiographs or reference table?**
A. Moyer's analysis
B. Hixson and Oldfather
C. Staley and Kerber
D. Tanaka and Johnson

160. **All the following cast analysis are used for evaluation of case for palatal expansion *except:***
A. Pont's index
B. Schwarz model analysis
C. BONN analysis
D. Bolton's analysis

161. **Which is the borderline case?**
A. If the arch length deficiency is 0-2.5 mm
B. If it is 2.5-5 mm
C. If it is more than 5 mm
D. None of the above

162. **Select one model analysis on lower permanent dentition:**
A. Carey's analysis
B. Ashley, How's analysis
C. Pont's Index
D. Moyer's analysis

157 D 158 C 159 D 160 D 161 B 162 A

163. On doing arch length analysis a discrepancy of 10 mm is noticed, treatment would be:
A. Expansion appliance
B. Proximal stripping
C. Orthodontic correction without extraction
D. Orthodontic correction with extraction

164. How do you preserve your patients study cast in the institution?
A. Photograph
B. Hologram
C. Preserving the study cast itself
D. All of the above

CEPHALOMETRIC ANALYSIS

165. Interincisal angle of 100° will indicate incisor:
A. Proclination
B. Retroclination
C. Normal position
D. None of the above

166. The Frankfort plane joins:
A. Nasion and Porion
B. Anterior nasal spine and pogonion
C. Porion and orbitale
D. Ala of nose and tragus

167. The most anterior part of bony chin is:
A. Gonion
B. Pogonion
C. Menton
D. Gnathion

168. A maxillary prognathism is indicated by a cephalometric SNA angle of:
A. 45° B. 67°
C. 84° D. 96°

163 D 164 B 165 A 166 C 167 B 168 D

169. Y axis in cephalometrics is a line joining:
A. Sella and Nasion
B. Gnathion and Menton
C. Gnathion and Orbitale
D. Sella and Gnathion

170. Which of the following cannot be assessed with cephalometric radiograph?
A. Mandibular retrusion
B. Maxillary retrusion
C. Mandibular lateral asymmetry
D. Incisor position and angulation

171. Normal IMPA angle is:
A. 100°
B. 90°
C. 80°
D. 70°

172. Negative ANB angle values indicate:
A. Class I malocclusion
B. Class II div 1 malocclusion
C. Class III malocclusion
D. Class II div 2 malocclusion

173. Normal interincisal angle is:
A. 110°
B. 105°
C. 90°
D. 132°

174. According to Tweed philosophy correct placement of these teeth is necessary to minimize relapse of:
A. Lower incisors
B. Upper incisors
C. Upper first molars
D. Lower first molars

175. SNA angle describes the relationship of the:
A. Maxilla to the cranial base
B. Mandible to the cranial base
C. Maxilla to the mandible
D. Maxilla to the upper incisors

169 D 170 C 171 B 172 C 173 D 174 A 175 A

176. Which of the following is a unilateral landmark?
A. Orbitale
B. Porion
C. Nasion
D. Gonion

177. High FMA angle leads to:
A. Deep bite
B. Open bite
C. Scissors bite
D. Cross bite

178. Angle of convexity:
A. SNA
B. SNB
C. N-A-Pog
D. ANB

179. Gonion, menton, pogonion are cephalometric landmarks located on:
A. Midline
B. Mandible
C. Bony chin
D. Profile skeletal

180. Y axis is used to analyse:
A. Maxillary growth
B. Mandibular growth
C. Both maxillary and mandibular growth
D. To design appliances

181. Which is the prognostic angle in 'Tweeds' analysis?
A. FMA
B. IMPA
C. FMIA
D. None of the above

182. The gonial angle at birth is:
A. 120°
B. 130°
C. 140°
D. 150°

176 C 177 B 178 C 179 B 180 B 181 A 182 B

183. Anthropometry deals with measurements:
- A. On dry skull
- B. On living individuals
- C. Landmarks established in studies of dry skulls are measured in living individuals
- D. All of the above

184. Facial angle is increased in:
- A. Class II malocclusion
- B. Class III malocclusion
- C. Class I malocclusion
- D. None of the above

185. The interincisal angle is increased in:
- A. Class I type 2 malocclusion
- B. Class II division 1 malocclusion
- C. Class II division 2 malocclusion
- D. Class III type 1 malocclusion

186. The Kesling diagnostic set-up of dental casts is related to the following angle on the lateral cephalogram:
- A. IMPA
- B. Y-axis angle
- C. FMIA

187. The most commonly used horizontal plane of orientation is:
- A. Sella-Nasion plane
- B. Occlusal plane
- C. Palatal plane
- D. Frankfort horizontal plane

188. An increased FMA in treatment planning signifies:
- A. Good prognosis
- B. Poor prognosis
- C. Has no relationship
- D. None of the above

---

183 C 184 B 185 C 186 C 187 D 188 B

189. The highest point on the concavity behind the occipital condyles is:
A. Bolton point
B. Glabella
C. Prosthion
D. Basion

190. On a profile cephalogram, porion is located at:
A. The highest point in the upward curvature of the retrocondylar fossa
B. The midpoint on the upper edge of the external auditory meatus located by means of ear rods on the cephalometer
C. The most posterior point is the concavity between pogonion and intradental
D. None of the above

191. If the norm for the cephalometric angle SNA is 82° a patient's reading of 90° of SNA most likely indicates:
A. Mandibular prognathism
B. Mandibular retrognathism
C. Maxillary prognathism
D. Maxillary retrognathism
E. Protrusive maxillary incisors

192. Cephalometrics is used in orthodontics to:
A. Treat malocclusion
B. Study growth changes
C. Aid in diagnosis and case analysis
D. All of the above
E. B and C
F. A and B

193. Key-ridge is:
A. A key for ridge expansion
B. The lowest point on outline of the zygoma
C. The lowest point on the angle of the mandible
D. Another name for SN plane

189 A 190 B 191 C 192 D 193 B

194. Cephalometry was introduced in 1934 by:

A. Hofrath in Germany
B. Broadbent in USA
C. Both of the above introducer
D. None of the above

195. Acanthion stands for:

A. Anterior nasal spine
B. Posterior nasal spine
C. Tip of anterior nasal spine
D. The point of intersection of the external dorsal contour of mandibular condyle and temporal bone

196. Bolton point is:

A. The most forward and lowest point on the anterior margin of the foramen magnum
B. Midpoint on a perpendicular from the sella to the Bolton-Nasion line
C. The lateral terminus of the oral slit
D. The highest point at the notches on the posterior end of the occipital condyles

197. The cranial base length is from:

A. Porion to Bolton point
B. Nasion to Bolton point
C. ANS to Bolton point
D. Acanthion to Bolton point

198. In standard cephalometric arrangement, the distance from the X-ray source to the subjects in mid-sagittal plane is:

A. 3 ft
B. 4 ft
C. 5 ft
D. 6 ft

199. The SN plane (Sella-Nasion) plane is oriented at:

A. 2 to 5° to FHP
B. 4 to 6° to FHP
C. 6 to 8° to FHP
D. 8 to 10° to FHP

194 C 195 C 196 D 197 B 198 C 199 C

200. In Cecil Steiner's analysis (1950), the magnitude of skeletal Jaw discrepancy is indicated by:

A. SNA angle
B. SNB angle
C. ANB angle
D. SN gonion angle

201. More than normal interincisal angle would indicate:

A. Bimaxillary protrusion
B. Open bite
C. Increased overjet
D. Deep bite

202. Superamentale on a cephalogram is:

A. Point A
B. Point B
C. Point Pog
D. Point Me

203. Cephalometric growth changes in a patient can be evaluated by superimposing on the:

A. FHP
B. S-N plane
C. Mandibular plane
D. Facial plane

204. Which is not the cephalometric analysis?

A. Steiner's analysis
B. Tweed's analysis
C. Bjork analysis
D. Carey's analysis

205. Clockwise rotation of mandible leads to:

A. Open bite
B. Cl-III
C. Cl-I
D. None of the above

206. Anti-Clockwise rotation of mandible leads to:

A. Deep bite
B. Closed bite
C. Open bite
D. Edge to edge bite

200 C 201 D 202 B 203 B 204 D 205 A

207. What is palatal plane?
A. A line joining ANS and PNS
B. A line joining Go and GN
C. A line joining SN – Point A
D. None of the above

208. How much angle should be between SN and GoGN?
A. 32° B. 28°
C. 35° D. 30°

209. In cephalometric analysis of children with malocclusion, the angle ANB is frequently used. In patients with severe class-II malocclusions this angle is:
A. Large
B. Small
C. Normal
D. Negative

210. Acceptable magnification on a cephalogram is:
A. 3 to 4%
B. 1 to 2%
C. 6 to 7%
D. 8 to 10%

211. On Ricket's esthetic plane, the lower lip:
A. Is 1 mm posterior to the plane
B. Is 1 mm anterior to the plane
C. Rests on the plane
D. Is 2 mm posterior to the plane

212. The angle of convexity with age:
A. Decreases in size
B. Increases in size
C. First increases upto 15 years and then decreases
D. Any of the above

213. High angle case is:
A. FMIA > 65° B. IMP > 100°
C. FMP > 35° D. SNA > 4°

---

206 A 207 A 208 A 209 A 210 C 211 C 212 A
213 C

214. A boy has ANB angle of -4° facial angle of 98°, he is a case of:

A. True Cl-III
B. Pseudo Cl-III
C. Skeletal class II
D. Dental class II

215. Which of the following tells about maxillomandibular relationship?

A. SNA
B. SNB
C. IMPA
D. ANB

216. The anatomic porion is:

A. The upper edge of the shadow of the auditory canal seen on cephalometric films
B. The location of radiopaque marker placed on the rod that extends into the external auditory meatus as part of the cephalometric head positioning device.
C. Difficult to locate
D. Reliable cephalometric landmark

217. The machine porion is:

A. The upper surface of the ear rod of the cephalometric headholder
B. The upper surface of the shadow of the auditory canal on the cephalogram
C. Not reliable cephalometric landmark
D. Difficult to locate

218. Which is preferred in modern cephalometrics to establish true horizontal plane?

A. Natural head position-NHP
B. Anatomic head positioning
C. Frankfort plane
D. SN plane

---

214 B 215 D 216 A 217 A 218 A

219. For diagnostic purpose, careful evaluation of facial proportion both in front and profile view is also known as:

A. Poor man's cephalometric analysis
B. Moyer's analysis
C. Bolton's analysis
D. Down's analysis

220. Which view of cephalogram is useful to diagnose facial asymmetry?

A. Lateral cephalogram
B. AP view
C. PA view
D. Lateral cephalogram in mouth wide open
E. None of the above

221. Gonial angle with age tends to:

A. Increase in size
B. Decrease in size
C. Increases upto 9 years and then decreases
D. Decreases upto 9 years and then increases

222. In a skeletal class III, the value of ANB will be:

A. 10
B. +2
C. +4
D. +6

223. Anteroposterior relation of jaws is measured by:

A. ANB angle
B. Angle between SN and FH plane
C. Angle between SN and mandibular plane
D. Facial angle

224. Sella turcica lies above:

A. Pons
B. Frontal sinus
C. Foramen ovale
D. Sphenoidal sinus

219 A 220 B 221 B 222 A 223 A 224 D

225. **Which of the following lines/planes represent the anterior cranial base?**
A. FHP
B. SN
C. Bolton plane
D. Occlusal plane

226. **Cephalometrics is useful in assessing which of the following relationships?**
A. Tooth to tooth
B. Bone to bone
C. Tooth to bone
D. All of the above

227. **The first cephalometric analysis which emphasize vertical and horizontal relationship and interaction between them is:**
A. Down's analysis
B. Sassouni's analysis
C. Steiner's analysis
D. Harvold's analysis

225 B 226 D 227 B

5

Etiology of Malocclusion

1. **Abnormal thick Labial frenum results in:**
   A. Midline diastema
   B. Imbrication
   C. Labial inclination of incisors
   D. Cross bite
2. **Commonest cause of midline diastema is:**
   A. Rotated canine
   B. Mesiodens
   C. Cleft palate
   D. Traumatic Occlusion
3. **If the maxillary deciduous central incisors are over retained, the permanent central incisors erupt:**
   A. Palatally
   B. Buccally
   C. Get transposed
   D. Get impacted
4. **The most common local cause of malocclusion is:**
   A. Hypothyroidism
   B. Presence of supernumerary teeth
   C. Early loss of primary teeth
   D. Late eruption of permanent teeth
5. **Prolonged thumb sucking directly results in all of the following *except:***
   A. Deep over bite
   B. Proclination of upper central incisors
   C. Rotation of upper laterals
   D. Constriction of maxilla

---

1 A   2 B   3 A   4 C   5 A

6. **The most typical presentation of a tongue thrust swallow is:**
   A. Deep bite
   B. Spacing
   C. Anterior open bite and spacing
   D. None of the above

7. **Lower anterior crowding develops due to:**
   A. Arch length deficiency B. Lack of Leeway space
   C. Lack of primate space D. All of the above

8. **Median diastema is caused by:**
   A. Abnormal labial frenum
   B. Peg-shaped lateral
   C. Supernumerary teeth
   D. All of the above

9. **One of the common causes of cleft lip and palate is:**
   A. Birth injury
   B. German measles during first trimester of pregnancy
   C. Uterine posture
   D. Abnormal foetal position

10. **Prolonged thumb sucking causes which of the following?**
    A. Torsoversion of teeth and crowding
    B. Anterior cross bite and posterior open bite
    C. Posterior cross bite and anterior protrusion
    D. Changes in the occlusion sufficient to allow the more potent deforming muscular forces to create full-fledged malocclusion

11. **Premature loss of deciduous maxillary second molar produces a malocclusion in the permanent dentition, characterized by:**
    A. A class II molar relationship on the affected side
    B. A class III molar relationship on the affected side
    C. A class I molar relationship on the affected side
    D. Delayed eruption of permanent molar

6 A 7 A 8 D 9 B 10 C 11 A

12. **"Pseudoanodontia" is a term used to describe:**
   A. Peg-shaped teeth
   B. Total absence of teeth
   C. Teeth present but do not erupt
   D. Partial absence of teeth

13. **'Hypothyroidism' is characterized by:**
   A. Constricted lower arch
   B. Short ramus and constricted maxillary arch
   C. Class III malocclusion and open bite
   D. B and C are true

14. **Thumb sucking in children over 4 years of age may lead to:**
   A. Open bite
   B. Open bite and retruded mandible
   C. Open bite and protrusion of maxillary teeth
   D. All of the above

15. **Malocclusion may lead to:**
   A. Dental decay
   B. Periodontal problems
   C. TMJ dysfunction
   D. All of the above

16. **Oligodontia stands for:**
   A. Congenital absence of all teeth
   B. Congenital absence of many but not all teeth
   C. Congenital absence of only few teeth
   D. None of the above

17. **Which of the following is not an etiology of malocclusion?**
   A. Genetic factors
   B. Supernumerary teeth
   C. Ectodermal dysplasia
   D. Lip sucking
   E. Gingival inflammation

---

12 C 13 D 14 C 15 D 16 B 17 E

18. The main cause of bruxism is:
A. Physiological problems
B. Periodontal problems
C. Traumatic occlusion
D. Psychological factors

19. Multiple supernumerary and unerupted teeth are the characteristic features of:
A. Treacher Collins syndrome
B. Ectodermal dysplasia
C. Cleidocranial dysplasia
D. Crouzon's syndrome

20. The most common aetiology of non-skeletal anterior cross bite is:
A. Delayed eruption of permanent teeth
B. Over retention of primary incisors
C. Lack of space for the permanent teeth
D. None of the above

21. 'Beta hypothesis' deals with:
A. Long-face syndrome and its allied problem
B. It is a terminology coined by Dunlap to break deleterious oral habits, in children who are amenable to reason
C. Deals with pressure resorption and deposition
D. None of the above

22. Which of the following statements is correct regarding the "submerged" primary molar?
A. Tooth is non-vital
B. The tooth is ankylosed
C. There is no permanent successor
D. Resorption of roots is not evident

23. Bottle feeding may be stopped in a child by the age of:
A. 6 to 12 months B. 12 to 18 months
C. 24 to 30 months D. 30 to 36 months

18 D 19 C 20 B 21 B 22 B 23 B

24. As compared to other anterior teeth, a maxillary canine is often found impacted because:
- A. It erupts at the corner position where the arch turns abruptly
- B. It is the last anterior tooth to erupt, leaving little space for it
- C. Shape and length of its root prevent its proper alignment
- D. Already·erupted premolars are mesially inclined

25. Nursing bottle caries is least likely to involve:
- A. Maxillary incisors
- B. Maxillary molars
- C. Mandibular incisors
- D. Mandibular molars

26. Cleft lip occurs due to disturbances in:
- A. 4 to 6 weeks of intrauterine life
- B. 6 to 8 weeks of intrauterine life
- C. 8 to 10 weeks of intrauterine life
- D. 10 to 12 weeks of intrauterine life

27. In thumb-sucking posterior cross-bite occurs due to:
- A. Loss of the normal outward thrust of the tongue
- B. Negative pressure within the oral cavity which causes
- C. A and B
- D. Loss of oral seal

28. If the maxillary central incisor is not erupted we must consider:
- A. Congenital absence
- B. Presence of a supernumerary tooth
- C. Eagle's syndrome
- D. None of the above

29. Which test is suitable to elicit mouth breathers?
- A. Butterfly technique
- B. On inspection
- C. On intra oral clinical examination
- D. None of the above

---

24 B 25 C 26 B 27 C 28 B 29 A

30. One significant intra-oral finding in mouth breather:
- **A.** Open bite
- **B.** Severe proclination of anteriors with deep bite
- **C.** Normal overjet and over bite
- **D.** None of the above

31. What is the throat problem the child has if she/he breaths through mouth?
- **A.** Adenoid problem
- **B.** Tonsil problem
- **C.** Combination A and B
- **D.** A or B

32. Which gland regress as the age advances?
- **A.** Adenoid
- **B.** Thyroid
- **C.** Tonsil
- **D.** Salivary gland

33. Peg shaped lateral cause:
- **A.** Midline diastema
- **B.** Esthetic problem
- **C.** Malocclusion
- **D.** Malrelationship

34. Who listed the characteristic of the infantile swallow?
- **A.** Moyers
- **B.** Enlow
- **C.** Kjelgren
- **D.** Nance

35. Which months the mature swallow characteristics are readily observable?
- **A.** 18 months
- **B.** 20 months
- **C.** 26 months
- **D.** Less than 18 months

---

30 A 31 C 32 A 33 A 34 A 35 A

36. **Tongue thrusting habit is often exaggerated by:**
   A. Enlarged tonsils
   B. Tongue-tie
   C. Cross bite
   D. Prognathic mandible

37. **Cleft lip and palate is:**
   A. Congenital
   B. Heredity
   C. Twin study
   D. Chromosomal disorder

38. **Supernumerary tooth is:**
   A. Congenital
   B. Heredity
   C. Dental anomaly
   D. Combination of A and B

39. **Midline diastema is due to:**
   A. Heredity
   B. Peg shaped lateral
   C. Tongue thrusting habit
   D. Supernumery teeth
   E. All of the above

40. **Which theory tells abnormal pressure habit?**
   A. Equilibrium theory
   B. Blood flow theory
   C. Learning theory
   D. Psychoanalytic theory
   E. Combination of C and D

41. **What is "Trident of habit factors"?**
   A. Duration, frequency and intensity
   B. Heavy, low and light pressure
   C. Intermittent, continuous and interrupted
   D. None of the above

36 A 37 A 38 C 39 E 40 E 41 A

42. **On an average swallowing occurs:**
    A. 500 times/day
    B. 600 times/day
    C. 700 times/day
    D. 800 times/day

43. **The facial profile of a mouth breather is typically:**
    A. Long and wide
    B. Short and wide
    C. Long and narrow
    D. Short and narrow

44. **Tongue thrusting habit may be accentuated by:**
    A. Prognathic mandible
    B. Deep bite
    C. Enlarged tonsils
    D. Cross bite

45. **Most commonly missing tooth in human dentition is:**
    A. Maxillary lateral incisor
    B. Maxillary second premolar
    C. Mandibular lateral incisor
    D. Mandibular second premolar

46. **A patient with Down's syndrome may have:**
    A. Microglossia
    B. Class II tendency
    C. Short anterior cranial base
    D. Proclined maxillary incisors

47. **Mouth breathing with enlarged adenoids and tonsils may be best described as:**
    A. Anatomic B. Obstructive
    C. Physiologic D. Habitual

48. **Mouth breathing can be:**
    A. Obstructive B. Habitual
    C. Anatomical D. All of the above

42 B 43 C 44 C 45 D 46 C 47 B 48 D

49. **Peg shaped teeth are commonly seen in:**
   A. Maxillary lateral incisor
   B. Mandibular lateral incisor
   C. Maxillary central incisor
   D. Mandibular central incisor

50. **Butterfly technique is adapted to elicit:**
   A. Mouth breathing
   B. Adenoid enlargement
   C. Tongue thrusting habit
   D. Abnormal swallowing habit

51. **Which syndrome is associated with cleft lip and cleft palate?**
   A. Trisomy 18
   B. Ectodermal dysplasia
   C. Van der Woude syndrome
   D. All of the above

52. **Which syndrome is associated with cleft palate alone?**
   A. Pierre Robin syndrome
   B. Apert syndrome
   C. Cleidocranial dysplasia
   D. All of the above

53. **Which clinical condition require the team work of pediatrician, plastic surgeon, orthodontist, oral surgeon and ENT surgeon?**
   A. Cleft lip and cleft palate
   B. Skeletal Cl-III cases after 14 years
   C. Long Face syndrome
   D. Sleep Apnea syndrome

54. **Teratogenic drugs like anti-convulsants and cortico-steroids lead to:**
   A. Cleft lip and cleft palate
   B. Facial palsy
   C. Facial deformity
   D. Mentally retarded growth of the child

49 A 50 A 51 D 52 D 53 A 54 A

55. **'Adenoid facies' is associated with:**
    A. Thumb sucking
    B. Tongue thrusting
    C. Mouth breathing
    D. Is a congenital anomaly

56. **Supernumerary teeth are found more commonly in:**
    A. Primary dentition
    B. Permanent dentition
    C. Mixed dentition
    D. None of the above

57. **Supernumerary teeth may give rise to:**
    A. Delayed eruption of teeth
    B. Malocclusion
    C. Dentigerous cysts
    D. All of the above

58. **Pierre Robin syndrome is characterized by:**
    A. Short mandible
    B. Enlarged tongue
    C. Cleft palate and short mandible
    D. All of the above

59. **The infantile swallow and suckling are well developed by about:**
    A. 28th week of IUL
    B. 30th week of IUL
    C. 32nd week of IUL
    D. 34th week of IUL

60. **Most children achieve most features of mature swallow at:**
    A. 10 to 12 months of age
    B. 12 to 15 months of age
    C. 15 to 18 months of age
    D. 18 to 20 months of age

---

55 C 56 B 57 D 58 D 59 C 60 B

61. **The characteristics of mature swallow include:**
   A. Teeth together swallow
   B. Mandible stabilize by 5th cranial nerve
   C. Tongue is held behind the incisor teeth and against the palate
   D. Minimum contraction of lip
   E. All of the above

62. **During mature swallowing, the mandible is stabilized by the:**
   A. 4th cranial nerve
   B. 5th cranial nerve
   C. 6th cranial nerve
   D. 9th cranial nerve

63. **A 9-year-old patient exhibits a lingually locked permanent maxillary left central incisor. Supporting bone is in harmony with tooth size and there are no basic discrepancies in other relationships. The most probable etiologic factor is:**
   A. Premature extraction of the primary maxillary right central incisor
   B. Prolonged retention of the primary maxillary left central incisor
   C. Premature extraction of the primary maxillary left central incisor with space loss in the area
   D. Pronounced facioversion on eruption of the permanent mandibular left central incisor

64. **Asymmetric anterior open bite with normal posterior occlusion is characteristic of:**
   A. Finger sucking
   B. Mouth breathing
   C. Abnormal swallowing
   D. None of the above

65. **Tongue thrusting habit in a 10-year-old patient is least likely to have caused:**
   A. Flaring of incisors
   B. Anterior open bite
   C. Incompetent lips
   D. Expanded upper arch

61 E 62 B 63 B 64 A 65 D

66. **Nuke Sauger nipples have been designed to prevent the problems of:**
A. Mouth breathing
B. Thumb sucking
C. Bruxism
D. Maxillary proclination

67. **Factors that influence malocclusion are all *except:***
A. Age
B. Sex
C. Race
D. Caries index

68. **In an otherwise normal 25 year-old individual with lower anterior crowding can be due to:**
A. Trauma
B. Proximal attrition
C. Impacted third molars
D. Late mandibular growth

69. **The cleft lip defect appears most commonly during:**
A. 5th to 6th week
B. 6th to 7th week
C. 7th to 8th week
D. 4th to 5th week

70. **Orofacial aberrations which extend beyond the teeth and include the maxilla, the mandible or both are termed as:**
A. Orthodontic anomalies
B. Eugnathic anomalies
C. Dysgnathic anomalies
D. Asymmetric anomalies

71. **The major etiologic factor responsible for Cl-II malocclusion is:**
A. Sleeping habits
B. Growth discrepancy
C. Thumb and tongue thrusting
D. Tooth to jaw size discrepancy

---

66 B 67 D 68 C 69 B 70 C 71 B

72. **The most common local cause of malocclusion is:**
A. Hypothyroidism
B. Presence of supernumerary teeth
C. Early loss of primary teeth
D. Late eruption of permanent teeth

73. **The facial profile of a mouth breather is typically:**
A. Long and wide
B. Short and wide
C. Long and narrow
D. Short and narrow

74. **The incidence of midline diastema in the maxillary arch is maximum at about the age of:**
A. 6 to 7 years
B. 10 to 12 years
C. 12 to 14 years
D. 14 to 18 years

75. **A heavy fibrous frenum is usually the cause of a midline diastema in the maxillary arch. At birth when no teeth are present this frenum:**
A. Runs along the alveolar ridge to insert into the incisive papilla
B. Is papery thin and thickens with age
C. Is yet to develop
D. Has a high attachment which is lowered with age

76. **Thumb sucking is normal upto:**
A. 2 months
B. 12 months
C. 3½ to 4 years
D. 12 years

77. **When do you start mechnotherapy to correct finger sucking habit?**
A. At 4 years
B. After 4 years
C. At 9 to 10 years
D. At 14 years

72 C 73 C 74 A 75 A 76 C 77 C

6

Biomechanics of Tooth Movement and Anchorage

BIOMECHANICS OF TOOTH MOVEMENT

1. **The type of forces exerted by removable functional appliance is:**
   A. Light continuous
   B. Heavy continuous
   C. Intermittent
   D. Interrupted

2. **Which of the following is most essential for orthodontic tooth movement to occur?**
   A. Completely developed root
   B. Vital tooth
   C. Cellular cementum
   D. Vital periodontal ligament

3. **An excessive orthodontic force used to move a tooth may cause the following reaction *except:***
   A. Hyalinization
   B. Undermining resorption
   C. Direct bone resorption
   D. Crushing of periodontal ligament

4. **Rotation correction is achieved by using:**
   A. Force through the center of rotation
   B. Force and a couple
   C. A couple
   D. Force passed away from the center of rotation

1 C 2 D 3 C 4 B

5. **Tooth movements in pulpless teeth compared to vital teeth is:**
   A. Slow
   B. Past
   C. Variable
   D. Same

6. **Which theory describes the tooth movement?**
   A. Equilibrium theory
   B. Pressure-tension theory
   C. Blood flow theory
   D. Combination of B and C

7. **Which is the ideal optimal orthodontic force for tooth movement?**
   A. 50 gm/sq.unit
   B. 20 to 26 gm/sq.unit
   C. 25 gm/sq.unit
   D. 100 gm/sq.unit

8. **Which of the following statements is true?**
   A. Force varies directly with the cube of the length of wire and inversely with the cube of the distance through which deflected
   B. Force varies inversely with the cube of the length of the wire and directly with the cube of the distance through which deflected
   C. Force varies directly with the cube of the length and the distance through which deflected
   D. Force varies inversely with the cube of the length and the distance through which deflected

9. **True bodily movement of a tooth can be obtained by applying force:**
   A. At the centre of rotation of a tooth
   B. On the incisal edge of the tooth
   C. At the centre of resistance of a tooth
   D. None of the above

---

5 D 6 D 7 B 8 B 9 C

10. **When a simple tipping force is applied to the crown of an incisor? The centre of rotation is usually located:**
    A. At the apex
    B. At the incisal edge
    C. At the cervical line
    D. One-third the root length from the apex
    E. Two-thirds the root length from the apex

11. **Cells responsible for bone resorption during orthodontic movement of teeth are:**
    A. Osteoblasts
    B. Odontoclasts
    C. Osteoclasts
    D. Pleuripotentional cells of the periodontal ligament

12. **The optimum force values to move an incisor are:**
    A. 100 to 150 gram
    B. 300 to 400 gram
    C. 50 to 70 gram
    D. 20- to 0 gram

13. **The rate of active tooth movement with removable expansion appliance should not exceed:**
    A. 0.5 mm/month
    B. 0.75 mm/month
    C. 1.00 mm/month
    D. 1.25 mm/month

14. **A 300 gm force is applied through a canine retractor, the following change will be noticed:**
    A. Hyalinization
    B. Rear root resorption
    C. Frontal root resorption
    D. Rapid tooth movement

15. **Width of the periodontal ligament in children is:**
    A. 0.25 mm B. 0.18 mm
    C. 0.3 mm D. 0.5 mm

---

10 D 11 C 12 B 13 C 14 A 15 A

16. **The major eruption mechanism is localized within the:**
    A. Periodontal ligament
    B. Lamina dura
    C. Cementum
    D. Both A and B

17. **The simplest form of orthodontic tooth movement is:**
    A. Tipping
    B. Rotation
    C. Bodily movement
    D. Intrusion
    E. Extrusion

18. **The force required for intrusion of incisor teeth:**
    A. 15 to 25 gm B. 25 to 50 gm
    C. 50 to 75 gm D. 75 to 90 gm

19. **The most efficient tooth movement is produced by application of following force by fixed appliance:**
    A. Light continuous force
    B. Heavy interrupted force
    C. Light intermittent force
    D. All of the above

20. **Intermittent orthodontic force is that:**
    A. Which declines slowly to zero between activation
    B. Decline abruptly to zero when the orthodontic appliances is removed by patient
    C. Force which maintains some fraction of applied force from one visit to the next visit
    D. None of above

21. **Which of the following tooth movement requires minimum amount of force?**
    A. Extrusion B. Tipping
    C. Rotation D. Bodily
    E. Root uprighting F. Intrusion

---

16 A 17 A 18 A 19 A 20 B 21 F

22. **The major theory of orthodontic tooth movement included:**
    A. Biological electricity, i.e. Piezoelectric theory
    B. Blood flow theory
    C. Both A and B
    D. None of the above

23. **Skeletal changes can be produced by application of force for a minimum hour/day:**
    A. 8 to 10 hrs/day
    B. 10-12 hrs/day
    C. 6-8 hrs/day
    D. 12-14 hrs/day

24. **The moment to force ratio for bodily movement of tooth M/F:**
    A. 4 : 6
    B. 6 : 8
    C. 8 : 10
    D. 10 : 12

25. **When the orthodontic force applied is light, resorption will probably be:**
    A. Apical
    B. Direct
    C. Indirect
    D. Undermining

26. **The amount of force required for tipping a tooth is:**
    A. 10 to 20 mm Hg
    B. 30 to 50 mm Hg
    C. 50 to 90 mm Hg
    D. 90 to 110 mm Hg

27. **A couple constitutes:**
    A. Two unequal, parallel forces acting in the same direction
    B. Two equal, parallel forces acting in the opposite directions
    C. Two unequal, non-parallel forces acting in the same direction
    D. Two equal, parallel forces acting in the same direction

---

22 C 23 A 24 C 25 B 26 B 27 B

28. **The first tissue to react when orthodontic forces are applied is:**
    A. PDL
    B. Cementum
    C. Dentine
    D. Alveolar bone

29. **During orthodontic tooth movement, periodontal ligament provides:**
    A. Osteoblasts
    B. Osteoclasts
    C. Both A and B
    D. None of the above

30. **The centre of rotation in bodily tooth movement is located:**
    A. Within the apical one-third
    B. At the junction of apical, and middle one-third
    C. At infinity
    D. Within the middle one-third

31. **In orthodontic treatment, rapid tooth movement will cause all *except:***
    A. Devitalisation of teeth
    B. Resorption of roots
    C. Diffuse calcification of pulp
    D. Ankylosis

32. **In primary tooth intrusion is common because:**
    A. Alveolar bone is pliable
    B. Vertical overlap of teeth
    C. Lip protection to maxillary anterior
    D. All of the above

33. **An orthodontic tooth movement that takes place along the vertical axis is:**
    A. Tipping B. Translation
    C. Intrusion D. Rotation

---

28 A 29 C 30 C 31 D 32 A 33 C

ANCHORAGE

34. **Anchorage is most effective in:**
    A. Round roots
    B. Flat roots
    C. Triangular roots
    D. Long roots

35. **During fixed mechanotherapy, a patient using class II elastics is utilizing:**
    A. Simple anchorage
    B. Baker's anchorage
    C. Reciprocal anchorage
    D. Intra-maxillary anchorage

36. **Unintended movement of anchor teeth is referred to as:**
    A. Stationary anchorage
    B. Simple anchorage
    C. Reciprocal anchorage
    D. Anchorage slippage

37. **An ideal example of stationary anchorage is:**
    A. Cervical anchorage
    B. Occipital anchorage
    C. Anchorage from forehead or chin
    D. All of the above

38. **Which of the following is related to reciprocal anchorage in orthodontic mechanotherapy?**
    A. Tipping force
    B. Extraoral force
    C. Bodily movement of a tooth
    D. Equal and opposite forces

39. **The type of anchorage in which two groups of teeth move in equal and opposite direction is called as:**
    A. Stationary B. Reciprocal
    C. Simple D. Compound

---

34 C 35 B 36 D 37 D 38 D 39 B

40. **Implants are used as anchorage control in orthodontics:**
    A. False
    B. True
    C. Partly correct
    D. Under research

41. **Which is the example for reciprocal anchorage?**
    A. Midline diastema correction
    B. Through the bite elastic
    C. Using Cl-II elastics
    D. Combination of A and B

42. **Which Law is applicable in anchorage?**
    A. Sir Issac Newton Law
    B. Canine Law
    C. Wolf's Law
    D. Coulomb's Law

43. **Which of the following is not a source of orthodontic anchorage?**
    A. Bone B. Root
    C. Dentine D. Skull

44. **Baker anchorage utilises:**
    A. Intermaxillary anchorage with screws
    B. Intramaxillary anchorage with screws
    C. Intermaxillary anchorage with elastics
    D. Intramaxillary anchorage with elastics

45. **Diastema closure involves:**
    A. Stationary anchorage
    B. Simple anchorage
    C. Reciprocal anchorage
    D. All of the above

46. **Occipital anchorage is related to:**
    A. Couple force B. Intraoral force
    C. Intramaxillary force D. Extraoral force
    E. Tipping force

---

40 B 41 D 42 A 43 C 44 C 45 D 46 D

47. **Stationary anchorage refers to anchor teeth which:**
   A. Are banded
   B. Cannot move
   C. Are not free to tilt
   D. Are supported by extraoral forces

48. **Anchorage in which the units in one jaw are used to effect tooth movement in the other jaw, is termed:**
   A. Intramaxillary anchorage
   B. Reciprocal anchorage
   C. Simple anchorage
   D. Intermaxillary anchorage

49. **An example of intermaxillary anchorage is:**
   A. Class-II elastics between maxillary and mandibular molars
   B. Intra-arch elastics
   C. Occipital headgear
   D. Retraction of maxillary anteriors by tipping them lingually using maxillary molars as anchorage

50. **Which of the following is an example of simple anchorage?**
   A. Intra-arch elastics
   B. Cervical headgear
   C. Diastema closure by tipping the crowns with elastic traction
   D. Bodily movement of molars in a mesial direction

51. **The type of anchorage in which the anchoring unit offers resistance to its bodily movement is:**
   A. Simple anchorage
   B. Stationary anchorage
   C. Reciprocal anchorage
   D. Intermaxillary anchorage

---

47 C 48 D 49 D 50 C 51 B

52. **Reciprocal anchorage is a term applied to:**
   A. High levels of forces between molar and central incisors
   B. Reciprocal movement of two teeth with the same periodontal area
   C. A force differential between cortical and medullary bone
   D. None of the above

---

52 B

7

Appliances

REMOVABLE APPLIANCE

1. **Which one of the following is the example of an auxillary spring?**
   A. Finger spring
   B. Z spring
   C. Canine retractor
   D. Apron spring

2. **Robert's retractor is used to:**
   A. Move molars mesially
   B. Move upper incisors palatally
   C. Move upper canines distally
   D. Move upper incisors labially

3. **The posterior bite plane is used in correcting:**
   A. Deep bite
   B. Anterior open bite
   C. Anterior cross bite
   D. Posterior cross bite

4. **The anterior bite plane should be trimmed so that it is:**
   A. Inclined at 15° to the occlusal plane
   B. Inclined at 30° to the occlusal plane
   C. Inclined at 45° to the occlusal plane
   D. Parallel to the occlusal plane

5. **The tongue blade is a simple device used for correction of:**
   A. Lip sucking
   B. Tongue thrusting
   C. Finger sucking
   D. Incisor cross bite

---

1 D 2 B 3 C 4 D 5 D

6. **Z springs are given to:**
   A. Expand the arch
   B. Move individual tooth labially
   C. Close midline diastema
   D. Move incisors palatally

7. **Robert's retractor is an example of:**
   A. Headgear
   B. Canine retractor
   C. Labial bow
   D. Coil spring

8. **High labial bow is made of:**
   A. 0.7 mm wire
   B. 0.4 mm wire
   C. 0.3 mm wire
   D. 1 mm wire

9. **Coffin spring can be used for:**
   A. Expansion
   B. Rotation
   C. Closure of midline diastema
   D. Correction of deep bite

10. **Buccal canine retractor is an example of:**
   A. Guided spring
   B. Self-supporting spring
   C. Auxillary spring
   D. Single coil spring

11. **Anchorage in a removable appliance is provided by:**
   A. Labial bow
   B. Finger springs
   C. Clasps
   D. Acrylic plates
   E. Combination of C and D

12. **Anterior bite plane is used to correct:**
   A. Cross bite
   B. Deep bite
   C. Open bite
   D. Tongue thrust

---

6 B 7 C 8 D 9 A 10 B 11 E 12 B

13. **Lip bumper is used:**
    - A. To move incisors inwards
    - B. To move molar distally
    - C. To move incisors labially
    - D. Combination of B and C

14. **Identify the screw used for total cross bite correction:**
    - A. Quad helix without modification
    - B. Three dimension expansion screw
    - C. Fan type expansion screw
    - D. Universal expansion screw

15. **Which of the following statements is true when a helical loop is used?**
    - A. The force is accordingly reduced but the range of force activity is increased
    - B. The force is accordingly increased but the range of force activity is decreased
    - C. Both the force and range of activity is decreased
    - D. Both the force and range of activity is increased

16. **A cantilever spring may be defined as a spring which is:**
    - A. Fixed at both the ends
    - B. Free at both the ends
    - C. Fixed at one end and deflected at the other beyond the elastic limit of the material
    - D. Fixed at one end and deflected at the other within the elastic limit of the material

17. **In scientific terms, the connection between the length, thickness and amount of deflection of a cantilever spring of round section is expressed by the formula:**
    - A. $D \alpha PL^3/T^4$
    - B. $D \alpha PL^4/T^3$
    - C. $D \alpha PL^4/PL^3$
    - D. $D \alpha PL^3/PT^4$

13 D 14 B 15 A 16 D 17 A

18. **In planning the distribution of clasps in an appliance, two well-placed and well-made clasps can ensure stability of an appliance. Which of the following statements is true?**
   A. A line drawn from a clasp on one side of an appliance to a clasp on the other side should pass through the centre of the appliance
   B. Two clasps place at the distal ends of the arch will permit an upper appliance to drop anteriorly
   C. Two clasps placed at the distal ends of the arch will permit the lower appliance to rise it easily
   D. Clasps should be about the centre of the buccal segments to induce greatest stability of an appliance
   E. All of the above

19. **Which of the following springs is used for expansion of the arch?**
   A. Finger spring
   B. Apron spring
   C. Z-spring
   D. Coffin spring

20. **A normal removable appliance in treatment of thumb-sucking habit is:**
   A. Hawley's appliance
   B. Activator
   C. Boley's appliance
   D. Crib

21. **Expansion screws produce an expansion of:**
   A. 2 mm per turn
   B. About 1 mm in each visit
   C. 1 mm expansion per half turn
   D. 0.25 mm per quarter turn

22. **When the diameter of a wire is doubled the force exerted on the teeth is:**
   A. 4 times
   B. ½ times
   C. 8 times
   D. 16 times

---

18 E 19 D 20 C 21 D 22 D

23. Vertical loops incorporated in each wire:
A. Increase its flexibility
B. Reduce the force exerted by the arch wire
C. Can be used to open spaces between crowded teeth
D. All of the above

24. One of disadvantage of removable appliance is:
A. Can be removed on socially sensitive occasions
B. Reduce chair time during initial stage of treatment
C. Allow some type of growth guidance
D. Treatment is heavily dependent on patient compliance

25. The "Split Plate" appliance was introduced by:
A. Martin Schwarz
B. Philip Adam
C. Edward H. Angle
D. George Crozat

26. The most effective retention device for removable appliance:
A. Adam clasp
B. Finger spring
C. Pin-head clasp
D. Ball clasp

27. A screw used for expansion of maxillary arch should under no circumstances be activated more than:
A. Twice a week
B. Thrice a week
C. Once a week
D. None of the above

28. All the split-plate appliances produce:
A. Only tipping movement
B. Only bodily movement
C. Both tipping and bodily movement
D. None of the above

23 D 24 D 25 A 26 A 27 A 28 A

29. The classic labial bow used in removable appliance was first designed by:
A. Charles Tweed
B. Charles Hawley
C. Philip Adam
D. George Crozat

30. The Adam clasp for molars and premolar is made of:
A. 0.6 mm wire
B. 0.7 mm wire
C. 0.8 mm wire
D. 0.4 mm wire

31. In Adam clasp, the angulation of the retentive points to the bridge portion of clasp should be:
A. 35° **B.** 40°
C. 45° **D.** 50°

32. Springs used for removable appliance should be fabricated from steel wire of:
A. Less than 0.5 mm wire
B. 0.5 mm wire
C. Has no relation with the diameter of wire used
D. None of the above

33. A major limitation of removable appliances is:
A. Inability to control root position
B. Treatment is heavily dependent on patient compliance
C. Can be removed on socially sensitive occasion
D. Has a fail safe effect

34. A patient wearing removable appliance should be seen at an interval at:
A. 2 to 4 weeks
B. 4 to 6 weeks
C. 6 to 8 weeks
D. 8 to 10 weeks

---

29 B 30 B 31 C 32 B 33 A 34 A

35. Posterior bite plane is contraindicated in:
A. Open bite
B. Bimaxillary protrusion
C. Deep bite
D. Functional retrusion

36. Maxillary arch expansion is least useful in:
A. Class I malocclusion
B. Class II malocclusion
C. Class III malocclusion
D. All of the above

37. An anterior bite plane does not aid in:
A. Increase in intercanine width
B. Inhibition of eruption of lower anteriors
C. Eruption of posteriors
D. Labial movement of maxillary incisors

38. Prolonged use of an anterior bite plane may lead to:
A. Retraction of maxillary incisors
B. Mesial drift of permanent molars
C. TMJ problems
D. Periodontitis

39. Which labial bow is used as a base for auxiliary spring?
A. High labial bow
B. Roberts retractor
C. Split labial bow
D. Extended labial bow

40. What is the other name of 3/4th clasp?
A. 'C' clasp
B. Full molar crib
C. Universal clasp
D. Arrowhead clasp

41. When the labial bow loop is passed between canine and 1st premolar on one side and on the other side between 1st premolar and 2nd premolar, it is called as:
A. Asymmetrical labial bow
B. Extended labial bow
C. Fitted labial bow
D. Long labial bow

35 C 36 A 37 D 38 C 39 A 40 A 41 A

42. **When there is no guide given for cantilever spring it is otherwise supported by:**
 A. Boxing
 B. No guide
 C. Using thicker wire
 D. Selecting some other spring

43. **The finger spring can be activated by:**
 A. Opening the coil
 B. Closing the coil
 C. Compressing the coil
 D. No activation

44. **The Robert's retractor is activated by:**
 A. Closing the Helix
 B. Opening the Helix
 C. Compressing the Helix
 D. No activation

45. **The labial bow loop is activated at frequent intervals of:**
 A. One week
 B. Two weeks
 C. Three weeks
 D. Four weeks

46. **How much activation is given for labial bow loop?**
 A. 0.5 mm
 B. 0.5 mm on each side of labial bow
 C. 1mm on each side of labial bow
 D. Less than 0.5 mm

47. **If the bridge of Adam's clasp is soldered with round tube, it is used in as:**
 A. Intra-oral appliance for head gear
 B. A retainer
 C. Means of engaging the elastics
 D. None of the above

42 A 43 A 44 A 45 B 46 B 47 A

48. Name any one of the clasp used on maxillary incisors:
- A. South end clasp
- B. Lingual clasp
- C. Eyelet clasp
- D. All of the above

49. Where is the location of short labial bow in case of tipping required?
- A. Junction between incisal third and middle third
- B. Incisal third
- C. Middle third
- D. Cervical third

50. How do you activate the helical canine retractor?
- A. By closing the coil
- B. By opening the coil
- C. By opening the coil, by cutting the free ends by one mm/activation and readapt
- D. Once adjusted and later no adjustment required

51. When a new maxillary removable orthodontic appliance is placed, the effect on the patient speech will probably include:
- A. Difficulty with linguoalveolar consonants for a few days
- B. Difficulty with lingual vowel for few days
- C. Difficulty with both linguoalveolar consonants and lingual vowel for several weeks
- D. No difficulty is found at all

52. Finger springs for removable appliance are best constructed using:
- A. Nitinol wire
- B. TMA wire
- C. Stainless steel wire
- D. Elgiloy wire

---

48 A 49 A 50 B 51 A 52 C

53. **How would you bond the wire to activate a correctly made palatal canine retractor?**
   A. Between the coil and its insertion into the base of the plate
   B. By opening out the coil
   C. Between the coil and the tooth but close to the coil
   D. Between the coil and the tooth but close to the tooth

54. **An appliance that helps in the correction of harmful oral habits by altering the afferent limb of the reflex is:**
   A. Retention appliance
   B. Functional appliance
   C. Habit breaking appliance
   D. Fixed appliance

55. **A whip spring used for the correction of a single tooth rotation is an example of:**
   A. Fixed appliance
   B. Semifixed appliance
   C. Retention appliance
   D. Functional appliance

56. **A patient of 6 years of age has unilateral cross bite due to functional shift of the mandible. The treatment of choice is:**
   A. Bilateral expansion of the maxillary arch
   B. Unilateral expansion of the maxillary teeth of affected side
   C. Unilateral expansion of the maxillary teeth of unaffected side
   D. No correction, but observation till the succedaneous teeth erupts

57. **If the posterior bite plane retains in the appliance for long time, what could be the adverse effect on the dental occlusion:**
   A. Supraeruption of upper/lower anteriors
   B. Change of occlusal table
   C. Development of deep bite
   D. All of the above

---

53 C 54 C 55 B 56 A 57 C

58. Which expansion appliance is suitable for cleft palate patients?
A. Niti expander
B. Rapid palatal expander
C. Slow type expander
D. Memory screw appliance
E. All of the above
F. None of the above

59. A canine retractor is a:
A. Closed end spring
B. Open end spring
C. Can function as both
D. None of the above

60. Which of the following is not a passive appliance?
A. Semifixed appliance
B. Functional appliances
C. Retention appliance
D. Habit breaking appliance

61. A canine retractor is a:
A. Closed end spring
B. Open end spring
C. Can function as both
D. None of the above

FUNCTIONAL APPLIANCE

62. The only Tissue borne functional appliance is:
A. Activator B. Bionator
C. Twin block D. Frankel

63. Contraindications of activator are all *except:*
A. High FMA
B. Growing period
C. Severely protruding maxilla
D. Severe crowding

58 E 59 A 60 A 61 B 62 D 63 B

64. **Oral screen is indicated in:**
   A. Retrognathic mandible
   B. Prognathic maxilla
   C. Mouth breathing habit
   D. Prognathic mandible

65. **Which is the full time wear removable functional appliance?**
   A. Monoblock
   B. Herbst appliance
   C. Twin block appliance
   D. Hyrax appliance

66. **A maxillary central incisor erupting in a lingually-directed path should be:**
   A. Corrected before it reaches the occlusal plane
   B. Allowed to erupt until all incisors can be banded
   C. Allowed to erupt into cross bite and then corrected
   D. Left as it is because the pressure of the tongue will correct it as it erupts

67. **In catalon's appliance, if the angle of inclined plane to the occlusal plane exceeds 45°, what could be the type of tooth movement?**
   A. Intrusion of incisor
   B. Extrusion of incisor
   C. Tipping
   D. Rotation

68. **What is the correct angle of inclined plane to the occlusal plane in catalons appliance?**
   A. 45° B. 60°
   C. 45° D. 60°

69. **What is the name of original clasp in Twin block appliance?**
   A. Adam's clasp B. Delta clasp
   C. Ball end clasp D. Triangular clasp

64 C 65 C 66 A 67 B 68 A 69 B

70. **Who is the inventor of Twin Block appliance:**
A. William Clark
B. Emil Herbst
C. Andrews
D. Wick Alexander
E. Anderson

71. **What is the total treatment time if incline plane is indicated?**
A. Two weeks
B. Three weeks
C. Four weeks
D. 10 days

72. **If the treatment is prolonged beyond the prescribed time in incline plane appliance, what could be the adverse effect on occlusion?**
A. Supra eruption of U/L posteriors changing the occlusal table
B. TMJ pain
C. Inability to eat
D. Muscle imbalance

73. **Point out one appliance which results shortest treatment time.**
A. Incline plane
B. Through the bite elastics in posterior cross bite
C. Midline diastema correction (6 mm space)
D. None of the above

74. **The fixed functional appliance used for the treatment of class II malocclusion in growing children:**
A. Twin-block appliance
B. Bionator
C. Anderson's activator
D. Herbst appliance

70 A 71 A 72 A 73 A 74 D

75. **The only tissue-borne functional appliance is:**
   A. Activator
   B. Bionator
   C. Twin-block
   D. Frankel

76. **One of the contraindications to the use of the functional appliance treatment is:**
   A. Class II malocclusion case with normally placed maxilla and retruded mandible
   B. Increased overjet and over bite
   C. Horizontal growth pattern of mandible (FMA $< 25°$)
   D. Mandibular dental protrusion

77. **A working bite for functional appliance in class II malocclusion is obtained with:**
   A. 4 to 6 mm mandibular advancement
   B. 3 to 4 mm posterior opening of mandible
   C. Edge to edge incisor bite
   D. Both A and B

78. **Monobloc is another name for:**
   A. Hawley's appliance
   B. Inclined plane
   C. Maxillary expansion appliance
   D. Activator

79. **An appliance that harnesses the natural forces and transmits it to the teeth and alveolar bone in a predetermined direction is:**
   A. Functional appliance
   B. Retention appliance
   C. Semifixed appliance
   D. Fixed appliance

80. **Mouth breathing can be corrected by:**
   A. Lip bumper
   B. Lingual arch
   C. Oral screen
   D. Hawley's appliance

75 D 76 D 77 D 78 D 79 A 80 C

81. **Which screw is used for Activator-III appliance?**
A. Norweigian screw
B. Fan type screw
C. Universal standard screw
D. Hyrax screw

82. **Which appliance is not suitable for skeletal Cl-III malocclusion at the age of 8 years?**
A. Frankel III
B. Activator III
C. Chin cap
D. Reverse pull headgear
E. Maxillary splint appliance

83. **A disadvantage of the activator is that it cannot:**
A. Help in correction of thumb sucking
B. Be used in cases with low facial height
C. Be used in skeletal maxillary protrusion
D. Utilize development during growth period

FIXED APPLIANCE

84. **The first appliance system designed by Angle was:**
A. Ribbon arch
B. E-Arch
C. Pin and tube
D. Edgewise appliance

85. **The straight wire appliance was developed from which of the following techniques?**
A. Begg
B. Edgewise
C. Ribbon arch
D. Tip edge

86. **The force needed to move teeth in a fixed appliance is derived from:**
A. Bands
B. Brackets
C. Archwires
D. Eyelets and cleats

81 A 82 E 83 A 84 B 85 B 86 C

87. Who is the father of straight wire appliance?
A. Andrews
B. Bennett
C. Wick Alexander
D. Begg

88. The edgewise appliance was introduced by:
A. PR Begg 1965
B. LF Andrews 1972
C. Edward Angle 1929
D. Johnson 1938

89. The apparatus used to measure the amount of pressure being exerted by a spring or elastic is known as:
A. Wanson Caliper
B. Vernier Caliper
C. Boley Gauge
D. Dontrix

90. The edgewise arch mechanism was introduced by Edward Angle in:
A. 1929
B. 1928
C. 1931
D. 1932

91. The following is not a component of fixed appliances:
A. Bands
B. Brackets
C. Open hellicie
D. Adam's clasp

92. Molar band material is normally:
A. 0.180 × 0.005 inch
B. 0.125 × 0.003 inch
C. 0.150 × 0.004 inch
D. 0.180 × 0.003 inch

87 A 88 C 89 D 90 A 91 D 92 A

93. **'Torque' in orthodontics indicates:**
   A. The change in mesiodistal inclination of teeth
   B. The change in labiolingual (axial) inclination of teeth
   C. The rotation of teeth
   D. All of above

94. **'Torque' can be applied to teeth by means of:**
   A. Twin-wire
   B. Laminated wire
   C. Rectangular wire
   D. Nitinol wire

95. **Intermaxillary elastics can be used in fixed and removable orthodontics for treatment of :**
   A. Class I malocclusion
   B. Class II malocclusion
   C. Class III malocclusion
   D. B and C

96. **The ribbon arch appliance was introduced by :**
   A. Mersnon B. Dewey
   C. Angle D. Tweed

97. **All the following appliances were introduced by Edward H Angle *except:***
   A. E. arch appliance
   B. Pin and tube appliance
   C. Edgewire appliance
   D. Straight wire appliance

98. **In Begg's technique, normally strategy for anchorage control is :**
   A. Tipping/uprighting
   B. Use of additional teeth within the same arch to anchor units
   C. Use of extraoral appliance (headgear) to first molar
   D. Use of transpalatal bar in upper arch and lingual bar in lower arch

93 B 94 C 95 D 96 C 97 D 98 A

99. **In straight wire appliance, all is true *except:***
   A. There is in-built provision in bracket for first order, second order and third order bends
   B. There is automatic rotational control mechanism
   C. A bracket slot dimension either 0.018″ × 0.030 ″ or 0.022″ × 0.030 ″
   D. It is a twin-wire appliance

100. **Followings are the indications for banding the teeth *except:***
   A. Teeth that will receive heavy intermittent forces against the attachments
   B. Teeth that will need both labial and lingual attachments
   C. Teeth with short clinical crowns which have incompatible surface for successful bending
   D. For aesthetic reasons

101. **The methods of separation of posterior teeth in orthodontic is:**
   A. Use of a brass wire
   B. Separating springs
   C. Elastomeric
   D. All of the above

102. **All is true for the tooth coloured or clear plastic brackets *except:***
   A. Tends to stain and discolours in mouth
   B. Less dimensionally stable than metal brackets
   C. Does not provide precise bracket slot
   D. It is very easy to slide the teeth to new position

103. **Most of preformed arch wire used in orthodontics is based on:**
   A. Bonwill-Hawley arch form
   B. Catenary curve
   C. Brader arch form
   D. Both B and C

---

99 D   100 D   101 D   102 D   103 D

104. Brackets with a rectangular slot are used in:
A. Edgewise technique
B. Begg's technique
C. Both
D. None

105. The width of a bracket is least decided by:
A. Width of the tooth
B. Convexity of the facial surface of the tooth
C. Shape and type of the archwire used
D. Rotational needs

106. Which of the following is least useful in correcting an ectopically erupting molar?
A. Separating device
B. Hawley's appliance
C. Brass wire ligature
D. Uprighting screws

107. One of the advantages of Direct Bonding technique:
A. Esthetics
B. Enamel crack
C. Staining
D. Decalcification

108. Methods of debonding the brackets:
A. Electrothermal debracketing
B. By debonding instruments
C. Laser debonding
D. All of the above

109. Application of magnets in orthodontic treatment:
A. Distalization of molar
B. Magnetic bracket
C. Canine impaction
D. All of the above

104 A 105 C 106 B 107 A 108 D 109 D

110. Which is the slow, continuous expander in maxillary arch?

A. Quad Helix
B. Niti expander
C. Hyrax
D. Norwegian screw

111. Who is the author of Herbst appliance?

A. Emil Herbst
B. Pancherz
C. Jasper Jumper
D. Edward Hartley Angle

112. Angle developed the following appliance:

A. 'E' arch
B. Edgewise appliance
C. Pin and tube appliance
D. Ribbon-arch appliance
E. All of the above

113. Which is the correct percentage of phosphoric acid for dull frosted appearance of etching?

A. 30% B. 30 to 36%
C. 35% D. More than 35%

114. What is the recommended time for etching in permanent teeth?

A. 30 to 60 seconds
B. 90 seconds
C. Less than 30 seconds
D. More than 90 seconds

115. How do you detect the proper etching clinically?

A. Dull frosted appearance of etched enamel
B. Smooth as enamel
C. Eroded
D. All of the above

---

110 B 111 A 112 E 113 C 114 A 115 A

116. If water or saliva contaminates with etched surface, what is the reaction on etched enamel?
A. Remineralisation takes place
B. Fluoride ions get absorbed
C. Less etching and poor bond strength
D. All of the above

117. Which is the esthetic bracket?
A. Ceramic brackets
B. Plastic brackets
C. Both A and B
D. None of the above

118. What is the choice of appliance suitable for skeletal Cl-II div.1 at the age of 14 years (Early permanent dentition)?
A. Herbst appliance
B. Twin block appliance
C. Either A or B
D. Fixed appliance

119. What is TPA?
A. Transpalatal arch
B. Treatment planning approach
C. Transverse plane articulation
D. None of the above
E. All of the above

120. Who demonstrated acid pretreatment in orthodontic practice?
A. Buonocore B. Miura
C. Retief D. Smith

121. How much percentage of phosphoric acid used by Buonocore in 1955?
A. 85% phosphoric acid
B. 65% phosphoric acid
C. 30% phosphoric acid
D. 36% phosphoric acid

116 D 117 C 118 C 119 A 120 A 121 A

122. Orthodontic brackets can be made up of all *except:*
- **A.** Stainless steel
- **B.** Gold
- **C.** Plastics
- **D.** Ceramics

123. Failure to upright a molar in an adult is usually due to:
- **A.** Lack of anchorage control
- **B.** Excessive force applied by the spring
- **C.** Stabilizing wire more active
- **D.** Occlusion not being relieved

124. Which is your choice of appliance if single molar is in cross bite?
- **A.** Through the elastics
- **B.** Expansion screws
- **C.** TPA (Transverse palatal arch)
- **D.** Niti expander

125. Sliding teeth along an arch wire would require at least a clearance of:
- **A.** 0.001″
- **B.** 0.002″
- **C.** 0.003″
- **D.** 0.004″

126. The etching agent in direct bonding technique contains:
- **A.** 15-30% unbuffered phosphoric acid
- **B.** 35-50% unbuffered phosphoric acid
- **C.** 35-50% buffered phosphoric acid
- **D.** 50-60% unbuffered phosphoric acid

127. As compared to indirect bonding technique, advantages of direct bonding technique include all *except:*
- **A.** Easier
- **B.** Faster
- **C.** Less expensive
- **D.** Provide accurate placement of bracket

---

122 B **123** A **124** A **125** B **126** B **127** D

128. Tooth positioner is a flexible rubber appliance used for:
A. Splinting of mobile teeth
B. Expansion of the arches
C. Correction of minor rotation/crowding by applying a passive force
D. Altering the frenum attachment passively to achieve a favourable tooth position

129. Correction of a posterior cross bite by using elastics is an example of:
A. Intermaxillary reciprocal simple single anchorage
B. Intermaxillary reciprocal simple compound anchorage
C. Intramaxillary reciprocal simple single anchorage
D. Intramaxillary reciprocal simple compound anchorage

130. Which of the following procedures is an example of corrective orthodontics?
A. Early elimination of oral habits
B. Fixed appliances
C. Mandibuloplasty
D. Planned serial extractions

131. The bond formed between a bracket and the enamel is:
A. Chemical
B. Mechanical
C. Ionic
D. Covalent

132. Orthodontic bands must:
A. Allow a thick layer of cement to be placed
B. Overextend on to gingival for esthetics
C. Have an inherent springiness to adapt well
D. Always be available in preformed shapes and sizes

133. A Siamese bracket is used in:
A. Begg's technique
B. Edgewise technique
C. Twin wire technique
D. All of the above

128 C 129 A 130 B 131 B 132 C 133 B

134. A semi-fixed appliance is:
A. An active appliance
B. A passive appliance
C. A retention appliance
D. An interceptive appliance

ORTHOPEDIC APPLIANCE

135. Orthopedic force is graded above the range:
A. 200 grams
B. 100 grams
C. 400 grams
D. 150 grams

136. Cervical pull headgear is indicated in:
A. Low angle cases with mandibular excess
B. High angle cases with mandibular excess
C. Low angle cases with maxillary excess
D. High angle cases with maxillary excess

137. Rapid palatal expansion is indicated in:
A. Anterior cross bite
B. Scissor bite
C. Bilateral posterior skeletal cross bite
D. Skeletal deep bite

138. The chin cap was introduced by:
A. Oppenhein
B. Sand steel
C. Cellini
D. Storey and Smith

139. Headgear tubes which are placed routinely on maxillary first molar for inner bow of face bow appliance are:
A. 0.045″ round tube
B. 0.051″ round tube
C. 0.052 round tube
D. Both A and B

134 A 135 C 136 C 137 C 138 A 139 D

140. Cervical headgear is contraindicated in:

A. Skeletal Class II base
B. Deep bite
C. Skeletal open bite
D. None

141. Which of the following appliances may cause molar extrusion?

A. Cervical head gear
B. High pull head gear
C. Chin cap
D. All of the above

142. What is the total treatment time if RME appliance is advocated?

A. 21 days
B. 15 days
C. 18 days
D. 20 days

143. In case of palatal expansion by RME appliance, the force advocated to separate the mid palatal suture is:

A. 2 to 3 pound
B. 3 to 5 pound
C. 5 to 7 pound
D. None of the above

144. A substantial increase in width of maxillary arch is best obtained by placing:

A. Lingual arch wire
B. Posterior intermaxillary cross-elastic (upper lingual to lower buccal)
C. A sutural expansion fixed appliance (RME)
D. A face-bow headgear with an expanded inner bow

145. The minimum force required to retard and redirect the maxillary growth:

A. 300 to 400 gm/side
B. 400 to 500 gm/side
C. 500 to 600 gm/side
D. 450 to 550 gm/side

---

140 C 141 A 142 A 143 C 144 C 145 A

146. The amount of force required to separate midpalatal suture in adolescence:
A. 1000 gm
B. 2000 gm
C. 3000 gm
D. 4000 gm

147. Use of extra oral force to move the maxilla forward is best done for children in the age group of:
A. 6 to 8 years
B. 8 to 10 years
C. 10 to 12 years
D. None of the above

148. The "infant orthopedics" was pioneered by:
A. Burston in Liverpool
B. Mc Namara
C. Emil Herbst
D. Andrews

149. The infant orthopedics is:
A. Orthodontic treatment for a newborn infant, before the eruption of any teeth
B. Feeding plate appliance
C. Niti expander
D. RME appliance

150. Who is ideal patient for chin cup?
A. One who has a mild skeletal problem, with the ability to bring the incisors end to end or nearly so
B. Pseudo Cl-III
C. True dental Cl-III
D. Severe skeletal Cl-III

151. Distalisation of molar is accomplished by:
A. Cervical headgear
B. Occipital headgear
C. Chin cap
D. All of the above

146 B 147 A 148 A 149 A 150 A 151 A

8

Preventive Orthodontics

1. **When lower 2nd deciduous molar is prematurely extracted before the eruption of permanent 1st molar what could be the choice of space maintainer?**
   A. Distal shoe appliance
   B. Bonded space maintainer
   C. Band and loop space maintainer
   D. Functional space maintainer

2. **The following conditions should be met by space maintainers:**
   A. Maintain the desired mesiodistal space
   B. Should not interfere with the eruption of the permanent tooth
   C. Should not interfere with the vertical eruption of the adjacent teeth
   D. All of the above

3. **The band and loop space maintainer is most frequently used:**
   A. To maintain in the space of a primary first molar before eruption of permanent first molar
   B. To maintain the space of permanent first molar
   C. For maintaining bilateral posterior space when more than one tooth is lost
   D. Both A and B

---

1 A 2 D 3 A

4. **If the mandibular second premolar is missing, then the primary second molar should:**
   A. Be extracted and space be maintained till the eruption of all permanent teeth
   B. Be retained if patient has an acceptable occlusion with slight mesiodistal grinding and later on replaced by fixed bridge
   C. Be extracted at an early age and be replaced by a fixed bridge
   D. None of the above

5. **In which of the following situations is space most difficult to manage?**
   A. A 9.5-year-old patient with loss of maxillary first molar
   B. A 5-year-old patient with loss of a primary maxillary central incisor
   C. A 6-year-old with loss of primary first molar
   D. A 5-year-old with loss of a primary mandibular second molar

6. **When multiple maxillary deciduous teeth are extracted bilaterally before shedding time, what could be your space maintainer?**
   A. Nance holding arch
   B. Lingual arch
   C. TPA
   D. Lip pumber

7. **When multiple mandibular deciduous teeth are extracted bilaterally before shedding time, what could be your space maintainer?**
   A. Nance holding arch
   B. Lingual arch
   C. TPA
   D. Lip Bumber

4 B 5 D 6 A 7 B

8. **When primary mandibular first and second molars are lost in an 8 years old patient, space is best maintained by constructing and placing:**
   A. Multiple space maintainers
   B. Bands on the remaining teeth
   C. A functional removable appliance
   D. A bilateral nonfunctional space maintainer

9. **A disadvantage of a removable space maintainer is that it:**
   A. Cannot be made esthetic
   B. Is difficult to keep clean
   C. Will not maintain vertical dimension
   D. May not be worn by the patient

10. **It is necessary to extract the primary mandibular second molar of a 4-year-old patient, which of the following retainers is indicated?**
    A. Band-loop
    B. Lingual arch
    C. Crown with a distal shoe
    D. Functional removable appliance

11. **A space maintainer is least needed if:**
    A. Permanent maxillary incisor is missing
    B. Permanent maxillary molar is missing
    C. Primary maxillary incisor is missing
    D. Primary maxillary molar is missing

12. **Arch perimeter is adversely affected due to premature loss of a primary second molar. A Nance arch space maintainer may be used if the loss has occurred:**
    A. Before the eruption of permanent first molar
    B. After the eruption of permanent first molar
    C. Before the eruption of the permanent central incisors
    D. After the eruption of the permanent central incisors

---

8 D 9 D 10 C 11 C 12 A

13. The steps taken to preserve the integrity of what appears to be normal at a specific time are included under:

A. Preventive orthodontics
B. Interceptive orthodontics
C. Corrective orthodontics
D. Surgical orthodontics

14. Which of the following steps is an example of preventive orthodontics?

A. Early recognition and elimination of oral habits
B. Planned serial extraction
C. Fixed appliance
D. Mandibuloplasty

15. Space maintainer is indicated:

A. When all primary teeth are present
B. When second premolar is already erupting
C. When second primary molar is lost before second premolar is ready to take its place
D. None of the above

16. Disadvantages of removable space maintainer are:

A. May be lost
B. May be broken
C. May irritate the soft tissue
D. All of the above

17. Fixed space maintainer used for bilateral loss of primary teeth in mandibular arch is:

A. Band and loop
B. Crown and loop
C. Band and bar
D. Lingual arch

18. Which of the following is an active space maintainer?

A. Band and loop
B. Lingual arch
C. Willets guiding shoe
D. Gerber's space regainer

13 A 14 A 15 C 16 D 17 D 18 D

19. What is reminder appliance?

A. Upper Hawley's appliance with beads in the tongue spike

B. Fixed habit breaking appliance

C. Fixed appliance with lingual cleats attached to lingual aspect of upper anteriors

D. None of the above

20. To regain arch length in the anterior segment by moving the incisors labially, one should:

A. Use a tongue blade

B. Use an inclined plane

C. Use a split-saddle acrylic space regainer

D. Evaluate the position of the teeth cephalometrically before beginning

21. Baby bottle syndrome can cause such severe destruction of the maxillary primary incisor that they will have to be removed. The major reason for replacement of these teeth via a fixed or removable appliance in the early primary dentition is:

A. Speech and esthetics

B. Form and function

C. Arch perimeter requirements in the transitional dentition

D. Incising and mastication

22. A 10-year-old patient has mandibular canines trying to erupt into a space insufficient by 2 mm. Primary second molars are large and firmly in space. First premolars are erupting. An acceptable preventive orthodontic procedure for this case would be:

A. Disking the mesial proximals of the mandibular primary second molars

B. Extracting the mandibular primary second molars

C. Placing a removable bite opener

D. Extracting the first premolars

---

19 A 20 D 21 A 22 A

9

Interceptive Orthodontics

1. **Who is the father of serial extraction?**
   A. Nance
   B. Andrews
   C. Bjork
   D. Edward Hartley Angle

2. **An 8-year-old boy exhibits premature loss of primary mandibular canines in an otherwise normal oral cavity. This condition is suggestive in:**
   A. Rootless primary canines in mandible
   B. Lack of oral hygiene methods
   C. Insufficiency in arch length
   D. Impaction of permanent mandibular lateral incisors

3. **Premature exfoliation of a primary canine may indicate:**
   A. An arch length deficiency
   B. An arch length excess
   C. Skeletal malocclusion
   D. All of the above

4. **In a serial extraction regime, removal of a deciduous canine does not:**
   A. Correct anterior cross bite
   B. Prevent mesial migration of permanent canine
   C. Prevent lingual eruption of lateral incisor
   D. Allow first premolars to erupt ahead of canine

5. **Serial extraction procedure are usually avoided in:**
   A. Premature loss of deciduous teeth
   B. Tooth size discrepancies
   C. Congenital absence of third molars
   D. Gingival recession of lower incisors

---

1 A 2 C 3 A 4 D 5 C

6. **Premature exfoliation of a primary canine may indicate:**
   A. An arch length excess
   B. An arch length deficiency
   C. A skeletal malocclusion
   D. None of the above

7. **The steps taken to recognize and eliminate potential irregularities and malposition in the developing dentofacial complex are included in:**
   A. Preventive orthodontics
   B. Interceptive orthodontics
   C. Corrective orthodontics
   D. Surgical orthodontics

8. **Which of the following steps is an example of interceptive orthodontics?**
   A. Early correction of proximal caries
   B. Planned serial extractions
   C. Removable appliance
   D. Semifixed appliance

9. **Interceptive and preventive orthodontics cannot be carried out after eruption of:**
   A. Second premolars
   B. First molars
   C. Second molars
   D. Third molars

10. **The usual regime followed in serial extraction is:**
   A. CD4
   B. 4DC
   C. DC4
   D. C4D

6 A 7 B 8 B 9 C 10 A

10

Surgical Orthodontics

1. **Which of the following statements is true?**
   A. Malocclusion requiring surgical correction should be undertaken before growth spurt is completed
   B. Malocclusion requiring surgical correction should be undertaken after growth spurt is completed
   C. Surgical correction of malocclusion has no relationship with active growth
   D. None of the above

2. **An 18-year-old boy's chin deviates to the right upon opening, which of the following is a possible cause?**
   i. Hyperplasia of the right condyle
   ii. Hyperplasia of the left condyle
   iii. Ankylosis of the left condyle
   iv. Ankylosis of the right condyle
   A. i and iii
   B. i and iv
   C. ii and iii
   D. ii and iv

3. **Treatment of cleft lip and palate:**
   A. The treatment is usually started for lip closure at 2 months of age
   B. Surgical closure of the palate is started at around 18 months – 2 years
   C. Orthodontics usually started after permanent teeth erupt and is of long duration
   D. The entire treatment is started at 3 ½ of age
   E. All of the above
   F. A, B and C are true

---

1 B 2 D 3 F

4. **Who discovered in 1950 the distraction osteogenesis?**
   A. Russian surgeon, Alizarov
   B. McNamara
   C. Jasper
   D. Clark

5. **Which is the major surgical orthodontic procedure?**
   A. Exposure of canine impaction and orthodontic treatment
   B. Therapeutic extraction
   C. Sagittal split osteotomy and fixed appliance
   D. All of the above

6. **Who is the good candidate for camouflage treatment?**
   A. Too old for successful growth modification
   B. Skeletal Cl-III cases or Cl-II cases
   C. Dental Cl-III cases or Cl-II cases
   D. None of the above

7. **Which is the correct age for orthognathic surgery?**
   A. Between 8 to 14 years
   B. After 14 years
   C. After 16 to 18 years
   D. At 20 years

8. **Labially impacted canine is brought orthodontically by means of:**
   A. Elastic chain attached the bracket on impacted canine to the main archwire
   B. Gold chain
   C. Attracting magnets
   D. All of the above

9. **Palatal canine impaction is best detected by:**
   A. Occlusal film
   B. Shift cone technique
   C. Mucosal bulging
   D. All of the above

---

4 A　5 C　6 A　7 B　8 D　9 D

10. **The envelop of discrepancy is applicable in surgical orthodontics:**
    A. Surgical orthodontics
    B. Interceptive orthodontics
    C. Preventive orthodontics
    D. Corrective orthodontics

11. **Surgical repair of a cleft palate done tightly may lead to the development of which malocclusion?**
    A. Angle's Class I
    B. Angle's Class II
    C. Angle's Class III
    D. Any of the above

---

10 A 11 B

11

Retention and Relapse

1. **No retention is needed in the treated cases of:**
   A. Mandibular crowding
   B. Anterior cross bite
   C. Midline cross bite
   D. Deep bite

2. **Relapse following orthodontic correction of rotation of teeth is associated with:**
   A. Supracrestal fibres
   B. Oblique fibres
   C. Horizontal fibres
   D. Diagonal fibres

3. **Supracrestal fibrotomy is done after correction of:**
   A. Crowding
   B. Proclined incisors
   C. Severely rotated teeth
   D. Space closure

4. **A corrected anterior cross bite is best retained by:**
   A. Over correction
   B. Retentive removable appliance
   C. Normal incisor relation
   D. Placing a Hawley retainer with palatal finger spring

5. **Recurring tooth rotations occur most frequently after orthodontic correction because of:**
   A. Density of the cortical bone
   B. Persistence of tongue and finger habits
   C. Persistence of free gingival and trans-septal fibres
   D. Persistence of oblique fibres of the periodontal ligament

---

1 B 2 A 3 C 4 C 5 C

6. **Fibers that are responsible for relapse of rotation movement of a tooth are:**
   A. Gingival
   B. Circumferential
   C. Oblique
   D. Horizontal

7. **Which retainer is ideal after midline diastema correction?**
   A. Bonded retainer
   B. Composite restoration
   C. Temporary retainer
   D. No retention

8. **Supracrestal fibrotomy is done to prevent relapse of a rotation movement of the tooth. Ideal retention period after surgery to allow new attachment of fibres is:**
   A. 8 weeks B. 12 weeks
   C. 16 weeks D. 24 weeks

9. **Which fibers are responsible for relapse?**
   A. Circular fibers
   B. Oxytal fibers
   C. Transseptal fibers
   D. All of the above

10. **How do you minimize the tendency of relapse in case of severe midline diastema after orthodontic correction:**
    A. Severing of Transseptal fibers
    B. Corticotomy followed by fixed appliance therapy
    C. Over correction
    D. Long period of retention
    E. Either or combination of above procedure

11. **Wrap around retainer's labial bow is attached to:**
    A. Adam's clasp
    B. 'C' clasp on the second molar
    C. Either A or B
    D. No attachment to any clasp. A single piece of wire is made as labial bow and finished around 2nd molar

6 B 7 A 8 C 9 D 10 E 11 C

12. **Which is active retainer?**
    A. After orthodontic treatment any minor correction can be carried during retention period
    B. It prevents the relapse
    C. It holds the corrected teeth in position
    D. None of the above

13. **The retention period for which the appliance is worn after completion of maxillary expansion is:**
    A. 1 month
    B. 3 months
    C. 5 months
    D. 9 months

12 A 13 B

12

Orthodontic Materials

1. **Passivating effect is due to formation of:**
   A. Iron oxide on austenitic steel
   B. Chromium oxide on stainless steel
   C. Bulky layer on polished acrylic
   D. Nickel oxide on martensitic steel
2. **Orthodontic wires and bands are made from:**
   A. Martensitic S.S.
   B. Austenitic S.S.
   C. Ferritic S.S.
   D. Carbon steel
3. **Which of the following orthodontic wire has shape memory phenomena?**
   A. Stainless steel
   B. Elgiloy
   C. Nitinol
   D. Composite plastic wires
4. **Which wire is ideal for coffin spring?**
   A. 19 gauge wire
   B. 22 gauge wire
   C. 21 gauge wire
   D. 30 gauge wire
5. **Which wire is used for unravelling the crowding?**
   A. Co-axial wire
   B. Niti wire
   C. Copper Niti wire
   D. All of the above

---

1 B 2 B 3 C 4 A 5 D

6. **Soldering and welding is not possible in:**
   A. Nitinol wire
   B. TMA wire
   C. Stainless steel wire
   D. Elgiloy wire

7. **Heat treatment for stainless steel wires can be done in an oven:**
   A. At 100°C for 5 minutes
   B. At 399°C for 10 minutes
   C. At 250°C for 10 minutes
   D. At 300°C for 10 minutes

8. **The most suitable material for fabrication of orthodontic springs is:**
   A. Nitinol
   B. 18-8 stainless steel
   C. β-titanium
   D. All of the above

9. **Heat treatment of stainless steel wires is done at low temperature in order to:**
   A. Increase modulus of elasticity and modulus of resilience
   B. Increase modulus of elasticity but decrease in modulus of resilience
   C. Decrease in modulus of elasticity but increase in modulus of resilience
   D. Decrease in modulus of elasticity and modulus of resilience

10. **The type of stainless steel with maximum corrosion resistance is:**
    A. Ferritic
    B. Austenitic
    C. Martensitic
    D. None

---

6 A 7 B 8 B 9 A 10 B

11. **The type of stainless steel with minimum carbon content is:**
    A. Ferritic
    B. Austenitic
    C. Martensitic
    D. None

12. **In order to dissolve the passivating film of chromium, flux used for stainless steels must contain:**
    A. Borax
    B. Boric acid
    C. Potassium fluoride
    D. Silica

13. **Titanium is added to stainless steel to:**
    A. Formation of a protective oxide layer
    B. Improve the resiliency
    C. Improve the strength
    D. Improve the hardness

14. **The solder for stainless steel wires contains:**
    A. Copper and silver
    B. Iron and copper
    C. Aluminium and iron
    D. Aluminium and silver

15. **In soldering technique, what is the role of antiflux?**
    A. Limits the flow of solder
    B. Remove the impurities
    C. Helps in good soldering
    D. Helps in avoiding voids in the soldered joint

16. **The nitinol wire does not have the property of:**
    A. Formability
    B. Springiness
    C. Strength
    D. Stiffness

---

11 B 12 C 13 B 14 A 15 A 16 A

17. Bending of loop is almost impossible with one of the following wires:

A. Nitinol wire
B. TMA wire
C. Stainless steel wire
D. Elgiloy wire

18. Which of the following wires is more useful in space closure and finishing?

A. Stainless steel wire
B. Nitinol wire
C. β-TMA wire
D. Elgiloy wire

19. The cement generally used for cementing orthodontic bands:

A. Zinc oxide cement
B. Glass ionomer cement
C. Zinc phosphate cement
D. Zinc silicophosphate cement

20. Elgiloy is:

A. Chrome cobalt alloy
B. Chrome gold alloy
C. Cobalt palladium alloy
D. Chrome palladium alloy

21. Thickness of the band material used in molars is:

A. 0.0003 inches
B. 0.03 inches
C. 0.005 inches
D. 0.05 inches

22. Thickness and width of bands used in the molar area is:

A. 0.005 x 0.180 inches
B. 0.005 x 0.150 inches
C. 0.005 x 0.125 inches
D. 0.05 x 0.150 inches

---

17 A 18 C 19 C 20 A 21 C 22 A

23. **Thickness and width of bands used in the premolar area is:**
    A. 0.04 x 0.150 inches
    B. 0.004 x 0.150 inches
    C. 0.005 x 0.150 inches
    D. 0.05 x 0.150 inches

24. **Brazing differs from soldering in that it:**
    A. Eliminates the use of flux
    B. Uses temperature above 450°C
    C. Is done with a gas air torch
    D. Applies to stainless steel wires only

25. **Doubling the cross section of wire, range of action:**
    A. Increases
    B. Decreases
    C. No effect
    D. First decreases and then increases

26. **All of the following materials have been used for orthodontic brackets** ***except:***
    A. Stainless steel
    B. White gold
    C. Plastics
    D. Ceramics

27. **All of the following may be applied to the tooth before placement of a bracket** ***except:***
    A. Composite
    B. Primer
    C. Etchant
    D. Fluoride gel

28. **If the passivating effect is lost in the orthodontic wire, what taste the child feels:**
    A. Metallic taste which is undesirable
    B. Better taste
    C. No taste
    D. None of the above

23 B 24 B 25 B 26 B 27 D 28 A

29. **The main form of iron carbide found in 18/8 stainless steel is:**
   A. Martensite
   B. Austenite
   C. Ferrite
   D. Pearlite

30. **Stainless steel is used most in dentistry:**
   A. To strengthen amalgam
   B. In orthodontic wires
   C. To construct clasps for partial dentures
   D. To replace internal gold restorations

31. **Which of the following wires is better choice if alignment is needed?**
   A. Nitinol wire
   B. TMA wire
   C. Stainless steel wire
   D. Elgiloy wire

32. **In Nitinol wire remember its shape in:**
   A. Austenite form
   B. Martensite form
   C. In both austenite and martensite form
   D. None of the above

---

29 B 30 B 31 A 32 B

13

Treatment Plan, Extraction and Superimposition

1. **A 7-year-old patient has a unilateral posterior cross bite due to a functional shift of the mandible. Indicated treatment involves:**
   A. Bilateral expansion of maxillary arch
   B. Unilateral expansion of maxillary posterior teeth on the affected side
   C. Unilateral expansion of maxillary posterior teeth on the unaffected side
   D. Muscle exercises to control shift of the mandible

2. **In a child with mixed dentition, it is not indicated to correct:**
   A. A transient class II malocclusion
   B. A class III malocclusion
   C. Thumb sucking habit
   D. All of the above

3. **A child who suffered from bilateral cleft lip and palate is brought to your clinic. Immediate treatment should be:**
   A. Posterior and anterior cross bite correction
   B. Expansion of mandibular arch which will cause maxilla to stretch
   C. Speech therapy
   D. Patient counseling and orthognathic surgery

---

1 A 2 A 3 B

4. **If the incisor overjet increases during treatment of a class-II div.1 case, you may be seeing:**
   A. Loss of anchorage
   B. Loss of retention
   C. Collapse of the lower arch
   D. Unfavourable growth

5. **The mother of a 10-year-old girl is concerned about a 1.5 mm diastema between the child's maxillary central incisors. A very fibrous maxillary frenum is present and inserts on the palatine papilla. When tension is applied to the frenum. The papilla blanches. The treatment of choice is to:**
   A. Perform a maxillary frenectomy to allow the teeth to close
   B. Close the space orthodontically expecting the frenum to atrophy due to pressure
   C. Postpone treatment until complete eruption of maxillary canines
   D. Close the space with a composite/veneer.

6. **Slow progress in molar uprighting in an adult patient is due to:**
   A. Overextended bands
   B. Lack of anchorage control
   C. The occlusion not being relieved
   D. The stabilizing wire not being passive

7. **Routine radiographic examination of a 6-year-old patient discloses a supernumerary tooth between maxillary central incisors. The dentist should:**
   A. Delay removal of the supernumerary tooth until its complete eruption
   B. Wait until the child is 12 years of age to remove the supernumerary tooth
   C. Remove the supernumerary tooth only if it develops acyst
   D. Remove the supernumerary tooth as soon as possible without injury to the central incisors.

---

4 A 5 C 6 C 7 D

Bibliography

1. Clinical Sciences – Dentogist MCQs in dentistry by Sanjeev Raj Bhatia, 2nd and 3rd editions.
2. Dental Examination Review by Atul Soin.
3. MCQs in Dental Sciences by Dhirendra Srivastava.
4. MCQs in Dentistry (Clinical Sciences) by Dr. Vijay Pratap Singh.